Statistics at Square Two

Understanding modern statistical applications in medicine

SECOND EDITION

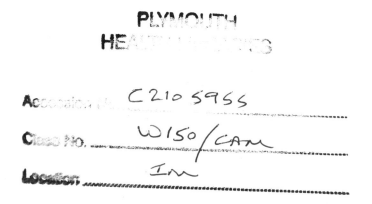

To David, John and Joseph

Statistics at Square Two

Understanding modern statistical applications in medicine

SECOND EDITION

Michael J. Campbell

Professor of Medical Statistics
University of Sheffield
Sheffield
UK

Blackwell
Publishing

© 2001 by BMJ Books
© 2006 M. J. Campbell

BMJ Books is an imprint of the BMJ Publishing Group Limited, used under licence

Blackwell Publishing, Inc., 350 Main Street, Malden, Massachusetts 02148-5020, USA
Blackwell Publishing Ltd, 9600 Garsington Road, Oxford OX4 2DQ, UK
Blackwell Publishing Asia Pty Ltd, 550 Swanston Street, Carlton, Victoria 3053, Australia

The right of the author to be identified as the author of this work has been asserted in
accordance with the Copyright, Designs and Patents Act 1988.

First published 2001
Second edition 2006

1   2006

Library of Congress Cataloging-in-Publication Data
Campbell, Michael J., PhD.
    Statistics at square two : understanding modern statistical applications
in medicine / Michael J. Campbell. — 2nd ed.
        p.   ;   cm.
    Includes bibliographical references and index.
    ISBN-13 : 978-1-4051-3490-3 (alk. paper)
    ISBN-10 : 1-4051-3490-9 (alk. paper)
    1. Medical statistics.   I. Title.
    [DNLM :   1. Statistics.   2. Biometry.   WA 950 C189s 2006]
    RA407.C36 2006
    610.2'1—dc22

                                                                        2006000620

ISBN-13: 978-1-4051-3490-3
ISBN-10: 1-4051-3490-9

A catalogue record for this title is available from the British Library

Set in 9.5/12pt Minion by Charon Tec Ltd, Chennai, India
www.charontec.com
Printed and bound in India by Replika Press Pvt. Ltd, Haryana

Commissioning Editor: Mary Banks
Development Editor: Nick Morgan
Production Controller: Debbie Wyer

For further information on Blackwell Publishing, visit our website:
http://www.blackwellpublishing.com

The publisher's policy is to use permanent paper from mills that operate a sustainable
forestry policy, and which has been manufactured from pulp processed using acid-free and
elementary chlorine-free practices. Furthermore, the publisher ensures that the text paper
and cover board used have met acceptable environmental accreditation standards.

Contents

Preface

When *Statistics at Square One* was first published in 1976 the type of statistics seen in the medical literature was relatively simple: means and medians, *t*-tests and Chi-squared tests. Carrying out complicated analyses then required arcane skills in calculation and computers, and was restricted to a minority who had undergone considerable training in data analysis. Since then statistical methodology has advanced considerably and, more recently, statistical software has become available to enable research workers to carry out complex analyses with little effort. It is now commonplace to see advanced statistical methods used in medical research, but often the training received by the practitioners has been restricted to a cursory reading of a software manual. I have this nightmare of investigators actually learning statistics by reading a computer package manual. This means that much statistical methodology is used rather uncritically, and the data to check whether the methods are valid are often not provided when the investigators write up their results.

This book is intended to build on *Statistics at Square One*.[1] It is hoped to be a "vade mecum" for investigators who have undergone a basic statistics course, to extend and explain what is found in the statistical package manuals and help in the presentation and reading of the literature. It is also intended for readers and users of the medical literature, but is intended to be rather more than a simple "bluffer's guide". Hopefully, it will encourage the user to seek professional help when necessary. Important sections in each chapter are tips on reporting about a particular technique and the book emphasises correct interpretation of results in the literature.

Since most researchers do not want to become statisticians, detailed explanations of the methodology will be avoided. I hope it will prove useful to students on postgraduate courses and for this reason there are a number of exercises.

The choice of topics reflects what I feel are commonly encountered in the medical literature, based on many years of statistical refereeing. The linking theme is regression models, and we cover multiple regression, logistic regression, Cox regression, ordinal regression and Poisson regression. The predominant philosophy is frequentist, since this reflects the literature and what is available in most packages. However, a section on the uses of Bayesian methods is given.

Probably the most important contribution of statistics to medical research is in the design of studies. I make no apology for an absence of direct design issues here, partly because I think an investigator should consult a specialist to design a study and partly because there are a number of books available.[2-5]

Most of the concepts in statistical inference have been covered in *Statistics at Square One*. In order to keep this book short, reference will be made to the earlier book for basic concepts. All the analyses described here have been conducted in STATA8.[6] However, most, if not all, can also be carried out using common statistical packages, such as SPSS, SAS, StatDirect or Splus.

While updating this book for the second edition, I have been motivated by two inclusion criteria: (i) techniques that are not included in elementary books but have widespread use, particularly as used in the *British Medical Journal*, the *New England Journal of Medicine* and other leading medical journals, and (ii) topics mentioned in the syllabus for the Part 1 Examinations of the Faculty of Public Health Medicine in the UK. I now have a section on what are known as *robust standard errors*, since they seem to me to be very useful, and are not widely appreciated at an elementary level. The most common use of random effects models would appear to be *meta-analysis* and so this is covered, including a description of *forest* and *funnel* plots. I have expanded the section on model building, to make it clearer how models are developed. *Simpson's paradox* is discussed under logistic regression. Recent developments in *Poisson regression* have appeared useful to me and so are included in the final chapter. All practical statisticians have to deal with missing data, hence I have discussed these and I have also added a Glossary.

I am also aware that most readers will want to use the book to help them interpret the literature and therefore I have removed the multiple-choice questions and replaced them with questions based on interpreting genuine papers.

I am grateful to Stephen Walters, Steven Julious and Jenny Freeman for support and comments, and to readers who contacted me, for making useful suggestions and removing some of the errors and ambiguities, and to David Machin and Ben Armstrong for their detailed comments on the manuscript for the first edition. Any remaining errors are my own.

Michael J. Campbell
Sheffield, 2006

Further reading

1. Swinscow TDV, Campbell MJ. *Statistics at Square One*, 10th edn. London: BMJ Books, 2002.
2. Armitage P, Berry G, Matthews JNS. *Statistical Methods in Medical Research*, 4th edn. Oxford: Blackwell Scientific Publications, 2002.
3. Altman DG. *Practical Statistics in Medical Research*. London: Chapman & Hall, 1991.
4. Campbell MJ, Machin D. *Medical Statistics: A Commonsense Approach*, 3rd edn. Chichester: John Wiley, 1999.
5. Machin D, Campbell MJ. *Design of Studies for Medical Research*. Chichester: John Wiley, 2005.
6. STATACorp. STATA Statistical Software Release 8.0. College Station, TX: STATA Corporation, 2003.

Chapter 1 **Models, tests and data**

Summary

This chapter introduces the idea of a *statistical model* and then links it to *statistical tests*. The use of statistical models greatly expands the utility of statistical analysis. The different types of *data* that commonly occur in medical research are described, because knowing how the data arise will help one to choose a particular statistical model.

1.1 Basics

Much medical research can be simplified as an investigation of an input–output relationship. The inputs, or explanatory variables, are thought to be related to the outcome, or *effect*. We wish to investigate whether one or more of the input variables are plausibly causally related to the effect. The relationship is complicated by other factors that are thought to be related to both the cause and the effect; these are *confounding factors*. A simple example would be the relationship between stress and high blood pressure. Does stress cause high blood pressure? Here the causal variable is a measure of stress, which we assume can be quantified, and the outcome is a blood pressure measurement. A confounding factor might be gender; men may be more prone to stress, but they may also be more prone to high blood pressure. If gender is a confounding factor, a study would need to take gender into account.

An important start in the analysis of data is to determine which variables are outputs and which variables are inputs, and of the latter which do we wish to investigate as causal, and which are confounders. Of course, depending on the question, a variable might serve as any of these. In a survey of the effects of smoking on chronic bronchitis, smoking is a causal variable. In a clinical trial to examine the effects of cognitive behavioural therapy on smoking habit, smoking is an outcome. In the above study of stress and high blood pressure, smoking may be a confounder.

However, before any analysis is done, and preferably in the original protocol, the investigator should decide on the causal, outcome and confounder variables.

1.2 Models

The relationship between inputs and outputs can be described by a mathematical model that relates the inputs, both causal variables and confounders (often called "independent variables" and denoted by x), with the output (often called "dependent variable" and denoted by y). Thus in the stress and blood pressure example above, we denote blood pressure by y, and stress and gender are both x variables. We wish to know if stress is still a good predictor of blood pressure when we know an individual's gender. To do this we need to assume that gender and stress combine in some way to affect blood pressure. As discussed in Swinscow and Campbell,[1] we describe the models at a *population* level. We take samples to get estimates of the population values. In general we will refer to population values using Greek letters, and estimates using Roman letters.

The most commonly used models are known as "linear models". They assume that the x variables combine in a linear fashion to predict y. Thus, if x_1 and x_2 are the two independent variables we assume that an equation of the form $\beta_0 + \beta_1 x_1 + \beta_2 x_2$ is the best predictor of y where β_0, β_1 and β_2 are constants and are known as *parameters* of the model. The method often used for estimating the parameters is known as *regression* and so these are the *regression parameters*. Of course, no model can predict the y variable perfectly, and the model acknowledges this by incorporating an *error* term. These linear models are appropriate when the outcome variable is Normally distributed.[1] The wonderful aspect of these models is that they can be generalised so that the modelling procedure is similar for many different situations, such as when the outcome is non-Normal or discrete. Thus different areas of statistics, such as t-tests and Chi-squared tests are unified, and dealt with in a similar manner using a method known as "generalised linear models".

When we have taken a sample, we can estimate the parameters of the model, and get a fit to the data. A simple description of the way that data relate to the model[2] is

$$DATA = FIT + RESIDUAL$$

The FIT is what is obtained from the model given the predictor variables. The RESIDUAL is the difference between the DATA and the FIT. For the linear model the residual is an estimate of the error term. For a generalised linear model this is not strictly the case, but the residual is useful for diagnosing poor fitting models, as we shall see later.

Do not forget, however, that models are simply an approximation to reality. "All models are wrong, but some are useful."

The subsequent chapters describe different models where the dependent variable takes different forms: continuous, binary, a survival time, and when the values are correlated in time. The rest of this chapter is a quick review of the basics covered in *Statistics at Square One*.

1.3 Types of data

Data can be divided into two main types: quantitative and qualitative. *Quantitative data* tend to be either continuous variables that one can measure (such as height, weight or blood pressure) or discrete variables (such as numbers of children per family or numbers of attacks of asthma per child per month). Thus count data are discrete and quantitative. Continuous variables are often described as having a Normal distribution, or being non-Normal. Having a Normal distribution means that if you plot a histogram of the data it would follow a particular "bell-shaped" curve. In practice, provided the data cluster about a single central point, and the distribution is symmetric about this point, it would be commonly considered close enough to Normal for most tests requiring Normality to be valid. Here one would expect the mean and median to be close. Non-Normal distributions tend to have asymmetric distributions (skewed) and the means and medians differ. Examples of non-Normally distributed variables include ages and salaries in a population. Sometimes the asymmetry is caused by outlying points that are in fact errors in the data and these need to be examined with care.

Note that it is a misnomer to talk of "non-parametric" data instead of non-Normally distributed data. Parameters belong to models, and what is meant by "non-parametric" data is data to which we cannot apply models, although as we shall see later, this is often a too limited view of statistical methods! An important feature of quantitative data is that you can deal with the numbers as having real meaning, so for example you can take averages of the data. This is in contrast to qualitative data, where the numbers are often convenient labels.

Qualitative data tend to be categories, thus people are male or female, European, American or Japanese, they have a disease or are in good health and can be described as *nominal* or *categorical*. If there are only two categories they are described as *binary* data. Sometimes the categories can be ordered, so for example a person can "get better", "stay the same" or "get worse". These are *ordinal* data. Often these will be scored, say, 1, 2, 3, but if you had two patients, one of whom got better and one of whom got worse, it makes no sense to say that on average they stayed the same! (A statistician is someone with their head in the oven and their feet in the fridge, but on average they are comfortable!). The important feature about ordinal data is that they can be ordered, but there is no obvious weighting system. For example, it is unclear how to weight "healthy", "ill" or "dead" as outcomes. (Often, as we shall see later, either scoring by giving consecutive whole numbers to the ordered categories and treating the ordinal variable as a quantitative variable or dichotomising the variable and treating it as binary may work well.) Count data, such as numbers of children per family appear ordinal, but here the important feature is that arithmetic is possible (2.4 children per family is meaningful). This is sometimes described as having *ratio* properties. A family with four children has twice as many children as one with two, but if we had an ordinal variable with four categories, say "strongly agree", "agree", "disagree" and "strongly disagree", and scored them 1–4, we cannot say that "strongly disagree", scored 4, is twice "agree", scored 2!

Qualitative data can also be formed by categorising continuous data. Thus, blood pressure is a continuous variable, but it can be split into "normotension" or "hypertension". This often makes it easier to summarise, for example 10% of the population have hypertension is easier to comprehend than a statement giving the mean and standard deviation of blood pressure in the population, although from the latter one could deduce the former (and more besides).

When the dependent variable is continuous, we use multiple regression, described in Chapter 2. When it is binary we use logistic regression or survival analysis described in Chapters 3 and 4, respectively. If the dependent variable is ordinal we use ordinal regression described in Chapter 6 and if it is count data, we use Poisson regression, also described in Chapter 6. In general, the question about what type of data are the independent variables is less important.

1.4 Significance tests

Significance tests such as the Chi-squared test and the *t*-test, and the interpretation of *P*-values were described in *Statistics at Square One*.[1] The usual format of statistical significance testing is to set up a *null hypothesis*, and then collect data. Using the null hypothesis, we test if the observed data are consistent with the null hypothesis. As an example, consider a clinical trial to compare a new diet with a standard diet to reduce weight in obese patients. The null hypothesis is that there is no difference between the two treatments in the final weight of the patients. The outcome is the difference in the mean weight after the two treatments. We can calculate the probability of getting the observed mean difference (or one more extreme), if the null hypothesis of no difference in the two diets were true. If this probability (the *P*-value) is sufficiently small we reject the null hypothesis and assume that the new diet differs from the standard. The usual method of doing this is to divide the mean difference in weight in the two diet groups by the estimated standard error (SE) of the difference and compare this ratio to either a *t*-distribution (small sample) or a Normal distribution (large sample).

The test as described above is known as Student's *t*-test, but the form of the test, whereby an estimate is divided by its SE and compared to a Normal distribution, is known as a *Wald test* or a *z-test*.

There are, in fact, a large number of different types of statistical test. For Normally distributed data, they usually give the same *P*-values, but for other types of data they can give different results. In the medical literature there are three different tests that are commonly used, and it is important to be aware of the basis of their construction and their differences. These tests are known as the *Wald test*, the *score* test and the *likelihood ratio test*. For non-Normally distributed data they can give different *P*-values, although usually the results converge as the data set increases in size. The basis for these three tests is described in Appendix 2.

1.5 Confidence intervals

The problem with statistical tests is that the *P*-value depends on the size of the data set. With a large enough data set, it would be almost always possible to prove that two treatments differed significantly, albeit by small amounts. It is important to present the results of an analysis with an estimate of the mean effect, and a measure of precision, such as a confidence interval (CI).[3] To understand a CI we need to consider the difference between a population and a sample. A population is a group to whom we make generalisations, such as patients with diabetes, or middle-aged men. Populations have *parameters*, such as the mean HbA1c in diabetics, or the mean blood pressure in middle-aged men. Models are used to model populations and so the parameters in a model are population parameters. We take samples to get *estimates* for model parameters. We cannot expect the estimate of a model parameter to be exactly equal to the true model parameter, but as the sample gets larger we would expect the estimate to get closer to the true value, and a CI about the estimate helps to quantify this. A 95% CI for a population mean implies that if we took 100 samples of a fixed size, and calculated the mean and 95% CI for each, then we would expect 95 of the intervals to include the true model parameter. The way they are commonly understood from a single sample is that there is a 95% chance that the population parameter is in the 95% CI.

In the diet example given above, the CI will measure how precisely we can estimate the effect of the new diet. If in fact the new diet were no different from the old, we would expect the CI for the effect measure to contain 0.

1.6 Statistical tests using models

A t-test compares the mean values of a continuous variable in two groups. This can be written as a linear model. In the example above, weight after treatment was the continuous variable, under one of two diets. Here the primary predictor variable x is Diet, which is a binary variable taking the value (say) 0 for the standard diet and 1 for the new diet. The outcome variable is weight. There are no confounding variables. The fitted model is Weight $= b_0 + b_1$ Diet + Residual. The FIT part of the model is $b_0 + b_1$ Diet and is what we would predict someone's weight to be given our estimate of the effect of the diet. We assume that the residuals have an approximate Normal distribution. The null hypothesis is that the coefficient associated with diet, b_1, is from a population with mean 0. Thus we assume that β_1, the population parameter, is 0. Thus, rather than using a simple test we can use a model. The results from a t-test and linear regression are compared in Appendix 3.

Models enable us to make our assumptions explicit. A nice feature about models, as opposed to tests, is that they are easily extended. Thus, weight at baseline may (by chance) differ in the two groups, and will be related to weight after treatment, so it could be included as a confounder variable.

This method is further described in Chapter 2 as multiple regression. The treatment of the Chi-squared test as a model is described in Chapter 3 under logistic regression.

1.7 Model fitting and analysis: confirmatory and exploratory analyses

There are two aspects to data analysis: confirmatory and exploratory analyses. In a *confirmatory analysis* we are testing a pre-specified hypothesis and it follows naturally to conduct significance tests. Testing for a treatment effect in a clinical trial is a good example of a confirmatory analysis. In an *exploratory analysis* we are looking to see what the data are telling us. An example would be looking for risk factors in a cohort study. The findings should be regarded as tentative to be confirmed in a subsequent study, and P-values are largely decorative. Often one can do both types of analysis in the same study. For example, when analysing a clinical trial, a large number of possible outcomes may have been measured. Those specified in the protocol as primary outcomes are subjected to a confirmatory analysis, but there is often a large amount of information, say concerning side effects, that could also be analysed. These should be reported, but with a warning that they emerged from the analysis and not from a pre-specified hypothesis. It seems illogical to ignore information in a study, but also the lure of an apparent unexpected significant result can be very difficult to resist (but should be)!

It may also be useful to distinguish *audit*, which is largely descriptive, intending to provide information about one particular time and place, and *research* which tries to be generalisable to other times and places.

1.8 Computer-intensive methods

Much of the theory described in the rest of this book requires some prescription of a distribution for the data, such as the Normal distribution. There are now methods available which use models but are less dependent on the actual distribution. They are very much computer-intensive and until recently were unfeasible. However, they are becoming more prevalent, and for completeness a description of one such method, the *bootstrap*, is given in Appendix 3.

1.9 Bayesian methods

The model-based approach to statistics leads one to statements such as "given model M, the probability of obtaining data D is *P*". This is known as the *frequentist* approach. This assumes that population parameters are fixed. However, many investigators would like to make statements about the probability of model M being true, in the form "given the data D, what is the probability that model M is the correct one?" Thus one would like to know, for example, what is the probability of a diet working. A statement of this form would be particularly helpful for people who have to make decisions about individual patients. This leads to a way of thinking known as "Bayesian", which allows population parameters to vary. This book is largely based on the frequentist approach. Most computer packages are also based on this approach. Further discussion is given in Chapter 5 and Appendix 4.

1.10 Missing values

Missing values are the bane of a statistical analyst's life and are usually not discussed in elementary textbooks. In any survey, for example, some people will not respond; at worst we need to know how many are missing and at best we would like some data on them, say their age and gender. Then we can make some elementary checks to see if the subjects who did respond are typical. One usually finds that the worst responders are young and male. One then has to decide whether anything needs to be done. For longitudinal data, it is important to distinguish values missing in the main outcome variables and values missing in covariates. For the outcome variables, missing values are often characterised into one of three groups: (i) missing completely at random (MCAR), (ii) missing at random (MAR) and (iii) not missing at random or non-ignorable (NI). The crucial difference between (i) and (ii) is that for (ii) the reason for a value being missing can depend on previously recorded input and outcome variables, but must not depend on the value that is missing. Thus a blood pressure value would be not missing at random (non-ignorable), if it was missing every time the blood pressure exceeded 180 mmHg (which we cannot measure but can say that it made the patient too ill to turn up). However, if it were missing because the previous value exceeded 180 mmHg and the patient was then taken out of the study then it may be MAR. The important point to be made is that the reason for missing in MAR is independent of the actual value of the observation *conditional* on previous observations.

In longitudinal clinical trials it used to be traditional to ignore subjects if the values were missing. However, this can lead to biased and inefficient treatment estimates. The usual method of dealing with missing values is called *last observation carried forward* (LOCF), which does exactly what it says. However, this can also lead to bias and a number of other techniques have been developed including *imputation*, where the missing value is guessed from other values. Multiple *imputation* gives a distribution of possible values and enables uncertainty about the missing values to be incorporated in the analysis. Care, thought and sensitivity analyses are needed with missing data. For further details see Little and Rubin.[4]

1.11 Reporting statistical results in the literature

The reporting of statistical results in the medical literature often leaves something to be desired. Here we will briefly give some tips that can be generally applied. In subsequent chapters we will consider specialised analyses.

For further information Lang and Secic[5] is recommended and they describe a variety of methods for reporting statistics in the medical literature. Checklists for reading and reporting statistical analyses are given in Altman *et al.*[3] For clinical trials the reader is referred to the revised CONSORT statement:[6]

- Always describe how the subjects were recruited and how many were entered into the study and how many dropped out. For clinical trials one should say how many were screened for entry, and describe the drop-outs by treatment group.
- Describe the model used and assumptions underlying the model and how these were verified.
- Always give an estimate of the main effect, with a measure of precision, such as a 95% CI as well as the *P*-value. It is important to give the right estimate. Thus in a clinical trial, while it is of interest to have the mean of the

outcome, by treatment group, the main measure of the effect is the difference in means and a CI *for the difference*. This can often not be derived from the CIs of the means for each treatment.
- Describe how the *P*-values were obtained (Wald, likelihood ratio or score) or the actual tests.
- It is sometimes useful to *describe* the data using binary data (e.g. percentage of people with hypertension) but *analyse* the continuous measurement (e.g. blood pressure).
- Describe which computer package was used. This will often explain why a particular test was used. Results from "home-grown" programs may need further verification.

1.12 Reading statistics in the literature

- From what population are the data drawn? Are the results generalisable? Was much of the data missing? Did many people refuse to cooperate? Was this investigated using a sensitivity analysis?
- Is the analysis confirmatory or exploratory? Is it research or audit?
- Have the correct statistical models been used?
- Do not be satisfied with statements such as "a significant effect was found". Ask what is the size of the effect and will it make a difference to patients (often described as a "clinically significant effect")?
- Are the results critically dependent on the assumptions about the models? Often the results are quite "robust" to the actual model, but this needs to be considered.

References

1. Swinscow TDV, Campbell MJ. *Statistics at Square One*, 10th edn. London: BMJ Books, 2002.
2. Chatfield C. *Problem Solving: A Statistician's Guide.* London: Chapman and Hall, 1995.
3. Altman DG, Machin D, Bryant TN, Gardner MJ, eds. *Statistics with Confidence*, 2nd edn. London: BMJ Books, 2000.
4. Little RJA, Rubin DB. *Statistical Analysis with Missing Data.* Chichester: John Wiley, 2002.
5. Lang TA, Secic M. *How to Report Statistics in Medicine: Annotated Guidelines for Authors, Editors and Reviewers.* Philadelphia, PA: American College of Physicians, 1997.
6. Altman DG, Schulz KF, Moher D, Egger M, Davidoff F, *et al.* The revised CONSORT statement for reporting randomized trials: explanation and elaboration. *Ann Intern Med* 2001; **134:** 663–94. http://w02.biomedcentral.com/content/pdf/1471-2288-1-2.pdf

Chapter 2 **Multiple linear regression**

Summary

When we wish to model a continuous outcome variable, then an appropriate analysis is often *multiple linear regression*. For simple linear regression we have one continuous input variable.[1] In multiple regression we generalise the method to more than one input variable and we will allow them to be continuous or categorical. We will discuss the use of *dummy* or *indicator variables* to model categories and investigate the sensitivity of models to individual data points using concepts such as *leverage* and *influence*. Multiple regression is a generalisation of the *analysis of variance* and *analysis of covariance*. The modelling techniques used here will be useful for the subsequent chapters.

2.1 The model

In multiple regression the basic model is the following:

$$y_i = \beta_0 + \beta_1 X_{i1} + \beta_2 X_{i2} + \cdots + \beta_k X_{ip} + \varepsilon_i. \tag{2.1}$$

We assume that the error term ε_i is Normally distributed, with mean 0 and standard deviation σ.

In terms of the model structure described in Chapter 1, the link is a linear one and the error term is Normal.

Here y_i is the output for unit or subject i and there are k input variables X_{i1}, $X_{i2}, \ldots, X_{ip}$. Often y_i is termed the *dependent* variable and the input variables $X_{i1}, X_{i2}, \ldots, X_{ip}$ are termed the *independent variables*. The latter can be continuous or nominal. However the term "independent" is a misnomer since the X's need not be independent of each other. Sometimes they are called the *explanatory* or *predictor* variables. Each of the input variables is associated with a *regression coefficient* $\beta_1, \beta_2, \ldots, \beta_p$. There is also an additive constant term β_0. These are the *model parameters*.

We can write the first section on the right-hand side of equation (2.1) as

$$LP_i = \beta_0 + \beta_1 X_{i1} + \beta_2 X_{i2} + \cdots + \beta_k X_{ip}$$

where LP_i is known as the *linear predictor* and is the value of y_i predicted by the input variables. The difference $y_i - LP_i = \varepsilon_i$ is the *error* term.

The models are fitted by choosing estimates $b_0, b_1, \ldots, b_p$, which minimise the sum of squares (SS) of the predicted error. These estimates are termed *ordinary least squares* estimates. Using these estimates we can calculate the fitted values y_i^{fit}, and the observed residuals $e_i = y_i - y_i^{fit}$ as discussed in Chapter 1. Here it is clear that the residuals estimate the error term. Further details are given in Draper and Smith[2].

2.2 Uses of multiple regression

1 To adjust the effects of an input variable on a continuous output variable for the effects of confounders. For example, to investigate the effect of diet on weight allowing for smoking habits. Here the dependent variable is the outcome from a clinical trial. The independent variables could be the two treatment groups (as a 0/1 binary variable), smoking (as a continuous variable in numbers of packs per week) and baseline weight. The multiple regression model allows one to compare the outcome between groups, having adjusted for differences in baseline weight and smoking habit. This is also known as *analysis of covariance.*

2 To analyse the simultaneous effects of a number of categorical variables on an output variable. An alternative technique is the *analysis of variance* but the same results can be achieved using multiple regression.

3 To predict a value of an outcome, for given inputs. For example, an investigator might wish to predict the forced expiratory volume (FEV_1) of a subject given age and height, so as to be able to calculate the observed FEV_1 as a percentage of predicted, and to decide if the observed FEV_1 is below, say, 80% of the predicted one.

2.3 Two independent variables

We will start off by considering two independent variables, which can be either continuous or binary. There are three possibilities: both variables continuous, both binary (0/1), or one continuous and one binary. We will anchor the examples in some real data.

Example

Consider the data given on the pulmonary anatomical deadspace and height in 15 children given in Swinscow and Campbell.[1] Suppose that of the 15 children, 8 had asthma and 4 bronchitis. The data are given in Table 2.1.

2.3.1 One continuous and one binary independent variable

In Swinscow and Campbell,[1] the question posed was whether there is a relationship between deadspace and height. Here we might ask, is there a different relationship between deadspace and height for asthmatics than for non-asthmatics?

Suppose the two independent variables are height and asthma status. There are a number of possible models:

1 *The slope and the intercept are the same for the two groups even though the means are different.*

The model is

$$\text{Deadspace} = \beta_0 + \beta_{\text{Height}} \times \text{Height}. \quad (2.2)$$

This is illustrated in Figure 2.1. This is the simple linear regression model described in Swinscow and Campbell.[1]

2 *The slopes are the same, but the intercepts are different.*

The model is

$$\text{Deadspace} = \beta_0 + \beta_{\text{Height}} \times \text{Height} + \beta_{\text{Asthma}} \times \text{Asthma}. \quad (2.3)$$

Table 2.1 Lung function data on 15 children

Child Number	Deadspace (ml)	Height (cm)	Asthma (0 = no, 1 = yes)	Age (years)	Bronchitis (0 = no, 1 = yes)
1	44	110	1	5	0
2	31	116	0	5	1
3	43	124	1	6	0
4	45	129	1	7	0
5	56	131	1	7	0
6	79	138	0	6	0
7	57	142	1	6	0
8	56	150	1	8	0
9	58	153	1	8	0
10	92	155	0	9	1
11	78	156	0	7	1
12	64	159	1	8	0
13	88	164	0	10	1
14	112	168	0	11	0
15	101	174	0	14	0

This is illustrated in Figure 2.2.

It can be seen from model (2.3) that the interpretation of the coefficient β_{Asthma} is the difference in the intercepts of the two parallel lines which have slope β_{Height}. It is the difference in deadspace between asthmatics and

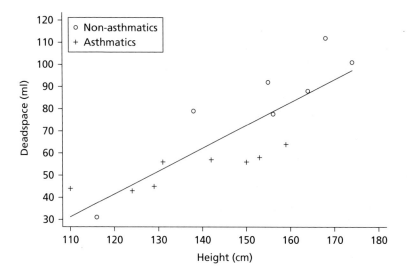

Figure 2.1 Deadspace vs height ignoring asthma status.

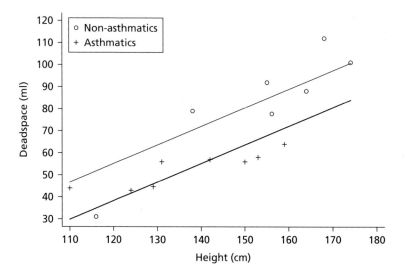

Figure 2.2 Parallel slopes for asthmatics and non-asthmatics.

non-asthmatics for any value of height, or in other words, it is the difference *allowing for* height. Thus if we thought that the only reason that asthmatics and non-asthmatics in our sample differed in the deadspace was because of a difference in height, and this is the sort of model we would fit. This type of model is termed an *analysis of covariance*. It is very common in the medical literature. An important assumption is that the slope is the same for the two groups.

We shall see later that, although they have the same symbol, we will get different estimates of β_{Height} when we fit equations (2.2) and (2.3).

3   *The slopes and the intercepts are different in each group.*

To model this we form a third variable $x_3 =$ Height $\times$ Asthma. Thus x_3 is the same as height when the subject is asthmatic and is 0 otherwise. The variable x_3 measures the *interaction* between asthma status and height. It measures by how much the slope between deadspace and height is affected by being an asthmatic.

The model is

$$\text{Deadspace} = \beta_0 + \beta_{\text{Height}} \times \text{Height} + \beta_{\text{Asthma}} \times \text{Asthma}$$
$$+ \beta_3 \times \text{Height} \times \text{Asthma}. \tag{2.4}$$

This is illustrated in Figure 2.3, in which we have separate slopes for non-asthmatics and asthmatics.

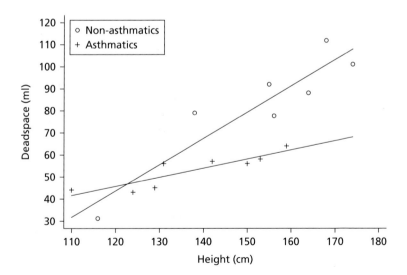

Figure 2.3 Separate lines for asthmatic and non-asthmatics.

The two lines are:
- *Non-asthmatics*
  Group = 0:

$$\text{Deadspace} = \beta_0 + \beta_{\text{Height}} \times \text{Height}$$

- *Asthmatics*
  Group = 1:

$$\text{Deadspace} = (\beta_0 + \beta_{\text{Asthma}}) + (\beta_{\text{Height}} + \beta_3) \times \text{Height}$$

In this model the interpretation of β_{Height} has changed from model (2.3). It is now the slope of the expected line for non-asthmatics. The slope of the line for asthmatics is $\beta_{\text{Height}} + \beta_3$. We then get the difference in slopes between asthmatics and non-asthmatics, which is given by β_3.

2.3.2 Two continuous independent variables

As an example of a situation where both independent variables are continuous, consider the data given in Table 2.1, but suppose we were interested in whether height and age together were important in the prediction of deadspace.
 The equation is

$$\text{Deadspace} = \beta_0 + \beta_{\text{Height}} \times \text{Height} + \beta_{\text{Age}} \times \text{Age}. \qquad (2.5)$$

The interpretation of this model is trickier than the earlier one and the graphical visualisation is more difficult. We have to imagine that we have a whole variety of subjects all of the same age, but of different heights. Then we expect the deadspace to go up by β_{Height} (ml) for each centimetre in height, irrespective of the age of the subjects. We also have to imagine a group of subjects, all of the same height, but different ages. Then we expect the deadspace to go up by β_{Age} (ml) for each year of age, irrespective of the heights of the subjects. The nice feature of this model is that we can estimate these coefficients reasonably even if none of the subjects has exactly the same age or height.
 If age and height were independent then we can reasonably expect the β_{Height} in equation (2.2) to be close to the β_{Height} in equation (2.5), but clearly in this case they are not.
 This model is commonly used in prediction as described in Section 2.2.

2.3.3 Categorical independent variables

In Table 2.1 the way that asthmatic status was coded is known as a *dummy* or *indicator* variable. There are two levels, asthmatic and non-asthmatic, and just one dummy variable, the coefficient of which measures the difference in the y variable between asthmatics and normals. For inference it does not matter

Table 2.2 One method of coding a three category variable

Status	x_1	x_2	x_3
Asthmatic	1	0	0
Bronchitic	0	1	0
Normal	0	0	1

if we code 1 for asthmatics and 0 for normals or vice versa. The only effect is to change the sign of the coefficient; the P-value will remain the same. However, Table 2.2 describes three categories: asthmatic, bronchitic and neither (taken as normal!), and these categories are mutually exclusive (i.e. there are no children with both asthma and bronchitis). Table 2.2 gives possible dummy variables for a group of three subjects.

We now have three possible contrasts: asthmatics vs bronchitics, asthmatics vs normals and bronchitics vs normals, but they are not all independent. Knowing two of the contrasts we can deduce the third (if you are not asthmatic or bronchitic, then you *must* be normal!). Thus we need to choose two of the three contrasts to include in the regression and thus two dummy variables to include in the regression. If we included all three variables, most regression programs would inform us politely that x_1, x_2 and x_3 were *aliased* (i.e. mutually dependent) and omit one of the variables from the equation. The dummy variable that is omitted from the regression is the one that the coefficients for the other variables are contrasted with, and is known as the *baseline* variable. Thus if x_3 is omitted in the regression that includes x_1 and x_2 in Table 2.2, then the coefficient attached to x_1 is the difference between deadspace for asthmatics and normals. Another way of looking at it is that the coefficient associated with the baseline is constrained to be 0.

2.4 Interpreting a computer output

We now describe how to interpret a computer output for linear regression. Most statistical packages produce an output similar to this one. The models are fitted using the *principle of least squares*, as explained in Appendix 2, and is equivalent to maximum likelihood when the error distribution is Normal. The estimate of the standard error (SE) is more sensitive to the Normality assumption than the estimate of the coefficients. There are two options available which do not require this assumption; these are the *bootstrap* and the *robust standard error*. Many computer packages have options for using these procedures. They are described in Appendix 3.

2.4.1 One continuous variable

The results of fitting model (2.2) to the data are shown in Table 2.3.

The computer program gives two sections of output. The first part refers to the fit of the overall model. The $F(1,13) = 32.81$ is what is known as an F-statistic (after the statistician Fisher), which depends on two numbers known as the *degrees of freedom*. The first, k, *is* the number of parameters in the model (excluding the constant term β_0) which in this case is 1 and the second is $n - p - 1$, where n is the number of observations and in this case is $15 - 1 - 1 = 13$. The Prob $>F$ is the probability that the variability associated with the model could have occurred by chance, on the assumption that the true model has only a constant term and no explanatory variables; in other words the overall significance of the model. This is given as 0.0001. An important statistic is the value R^2, which is the proportion of variance of the original data explained by the model and in this model it is 0.7162. It is the ratio of the sum of squares (SS) due to the model (5607) and the total SS (7828). For models with only one independent variable, as in this case, it is simply the square of the correlation coefficient described in Swinscow and Campbell.[1] However, one can always obtain an arbitrarily good fit by fitting as many parameters as there are observations. To allow for this, we calculate the R^2 *adjusted for degrees of freedom*, which is $R_a^2 = 1 - (1 - R^2)(n - 1)/(n - p - 1)$ and in this case is given by 0.6944. The Root MSE means the Residual Mean Square Error and has the value 13.072. It is an estimate of σ in equation (2.1), and can be deduced as the square root of the residual MS (mean square) on the left-hand side of the table. Thus $\sqrt{170.8847} = 13.072$.

The second part examines the coefficients in the model. The slope $\beta_{\text{Height}} = 1.0333$ and suggests that if one person was 1 cm taller than another we would expect their deadspace to be about 1 ml greater (perhaps easier to think

Table 2.3 Output from computer program fitting height to deadspace for data from Table 2.1

Source	SS	df	MS				Number of obs	=	15
Model	5607.43156	1	5607.43156				F(1, 13)	=	32.81
Residual	2221.50178	13	170.884752				Prob > F	=	0.0001
							R-squared	=	0.7162
							Adj R-squared	=	0.6944
Total	7828.93333	14	559.209524				Root MSE	=	13.072

Deadspace	Coef.	Std. Err.	t	P>|t|	[95% Conf. Interval]	
Height	1.033323	.1803872	5.73	0.000	.6436202	1.423026
_cons	-82.4852	26.30147	-3.14	0.008	-139.3061	-25.66433

if one person were 10 cm taller their deadspace is expected to be 10 ml greater). It is the slope of the line in Figure 2.1. The intercept $\beta_0 = -82.4582$. This is the value when the line cuts the x-axis when $x = 0$ (not the axis on the figure which is at $x = 110$). This is the predicted value of deadspace for someone with no height and is clearly a nonsense value. However, the parameter is necessary for correct interpretation of the model. Note these values are derived directly in Swinscow and Campbell (Chapter 11 in *Statistics at Square One*, 10th edn).

2.4.2 One continuous variable and one binary independent variable

We must first create a new variable Asthma = 1 for asthmatics and Asthma = 0 for non-asthmatics. This gives model (2.2), and the results of fitting this model are shown in Table 2.4.

In the top part of the output, the F-statistic now has 2 and 12 d.f., because we are fitting two independent variables. The P-value is given as 0.0000, which we interpret as <0.0001. It means that fitting both variables *simultaneously* gives a highly significant fit. It does *not* tell us about individual variables. One can see that the adjusted R^2 is greater and the Root MSE is smaller than that in Table 2.3, indicating a better fitting model than model (2.2).

In the bottom part of the output the coefficient associated with height is $\beta_{\text{Height}} = 0.845$, which is less than the same coefficient in Table 2.3. It is the slope of each of the parallel lines in Figure 2.2. It can be seen that because non-asthmatics have a higher deadspace forcing a single line through the data gives a greater slope. The vertical distance between the two lines is the coefficient associated with asthma, $\beta_{\text{Asthma}} = -16.81$. As we coded asthma as 1

Table 2.4 Output from computer program fitting height and asthma to deadspace from Table 2.1

Source	SS	df	MS			
				Number of obs	=	15
				F(2, 12)	=	28.74
Model	6476.91571	2	3238.45785	Prob > F	=	0.0000
Residual	1352.01763	12	112.668136	R-squared	=	0.8273
				Adj R-squared	=	0.7985
Total	7828.93333	14	559.209524	Root MSE	=	10.615

Deadspace	Coef.	Std. Err.	t	P>|t|	[95% Conf.	Interval]
Height	.8450468	.1613921	5.24	0.000	.4934035	1.19669
Asthma	-16.81551	6.053128	-2.78	0.017	-30.00414	-3.626881
_cons	-46.29216	25.01679	-1.85	0.089	-100.7991	8.214733

and non-asthma as 0, the negative sign indicates asthmatics have a lower deadspace for a given height.

2.4.3 One continuous variable and one binary independent variable with their interaction

We now create a new variable AsthmaHt = Asthma × Height for the interaction of asthma and height. Some packages can do both of these automatically if one declares asthma as a "factor" or as "categorical", and fits a term such as "Asthma*Height" to give model (2.4).

The results of fitting these variables using a computer program are given in Table 2.5.

We fit three independent variables: Height, Asthma and AsthmaHt on Deadspace. This is equivalent to model (2.4), and is shown in Figure 2.3. Now $F(3,11) = 37.08$ and $R^2 = 0.91$, the R^2 adjusted for d.f. is given by 0.89 which is an improvement on model (2.3). The Root MSE has the value 8.0031, which again indicates an improvement on the earlier model.

In the second part of the output we see that the interaction term between height and asthma status is significant ($P = 0.009$). The *difference* in the slopes is −0.778 units (95% CI −1.317 to −0.240). There are no terms to drop from the model. Note, even if one of the main terms, asthma or height was not significant, we would *not* drop it from the model if the interaction was significant, since the interaction cannot be interpreted in the absence of the main effects, which in this case are asthma and height.

The two lines of best fit are:

Non-asthmatics:

$$\text{Deadspace} = -99.46 + 1.193 \times \text{Height}$$

Table 2.5 Output from computer program fitting height and asthma status and their interaction to deadspace from Table 2.1

Source	SS	df	MS		Number of obs	=	15
					F(3, 11)	=	37.08
Model	7124.3865	3	2374.7955		Prob > F	=	0.0000
Residual	704.546834	11	64.0497122		R-squared	=	0.9100
					Adj R-squared	=	0.8855
Total	7828.93333	14	559.209524		Root MSE	=	8.0031

Deadspace	Coef.	Std. Err.	t	P>|t|	[95% Conf.	Interval]
Height	1.192565	.1635673	7.291	0.000	.8325555	1.552574
Asthma	95.47263	35.61056	2.681	0.021	17.09433	173.8509
AsthmaHt	-.7782494	.2447751	-3.179	0.009	-1.316996	-.239503
_cons	-99.46241	25.20795	-3.946	0.002	-154.9447	-43.98009

Asthmatics:

$$\text{Deadspace} = (-99.46 + 95.47) + (1.193 - 0.778) \times \text{Height}$$
$$= -3.99 + 0.415 \times \text{Height}$$

Thus the deadspace in asthmatics appears to grow more slowly with height than that of non-asthmatics.

This is the best fit model for the data. Using model (2.2) or (2.3) for prediction, say, would result in a greater error. It is important, when considering which is the best model to look at the R^2 adjusted as well as the P-values. Sometimes a term can be added that gives a significant P-value, but only a marginal improvement in R^2 adjusted, and for the sake of simplicity may not be included as the best model.

2.4.4 Two independent variables: both continuous

Here we were interested in whether height or age or both were important in the prediction of deadspace. The analysis is given in Table 2.6.

The equation is

$$\text{Deadspace} = -59.05 + 0.707 \times \text{Height} + 3.045 \times \text{Age}.$$

The interpretation of this model is described in Section 2.3.2. Note a peculiar feature of this output. Although the overall model is significant ($P = 0.0003$) neither of the coefficients associated with height and age are significant ($P = 0.063$ and 0.291, respectively)! This occurs because age and height are strongly correlated, and highlights the importance of looking at the overall fit of a model. Dropping either will leave the other as a significant predictor in the model. Note that if we drop age, the adjusted R^2 is not greatly affected ($R^2 = 0.6944$ for height alone compared to 0.6995 for age and height) suggesting that height is a better predictor.

Table 2.6 Output from computer program fitting age and height to deadspace from Table 2.1

Source	SS	df	MS			
Model	5812.17397	2	2906.08698	Number of obs	=	15
Residual	2016.75936	12	168.06328	F(2, 12)	=	17.29
				Prob > F	=	0.0003
				R-squared	=	0.7424
Total	7828.93333	14	559.209524	Adj R-squared	=	0.6995
				Root MSE	=	12.964

Deadspace	Coef.	Std. Err.	t	P>|t|	[95% Conf. Interval]	
Height	.7070318	.3455362	2.046	0.063	-.0458268	1.45989
Age	3.044691	2.758517	1.104	0.291	-2.965602	9.054984
_cons	-59.05205	33.63162	-1.756	0.105	-132.329	14.22495

2.4.5 Categorical independent variables

It will help the interpretation in this section to know that the mean values (ml) for deadspace for the three groups are normals 97.33, asthmatics 52.88 and bronchitics 72.25.

The analysis is given in the first half of Table 2.7. Here the two independent variables are x_1 and x_2 (refer to Table 2.2). As we noted before an important point to check is that, in general, one should see that the overall model is significant, before looking at the individual contrasts. Here we have Prob > $F = 0.0063$, which means that the overall model is highly significant. If we look at the individual contrasts we see that the coefficient associated with asthma -44.46 is the difference in means between normals and asthmatics. This has a SE of 11.33 and so is highly significant. The coefficient associated with bronchitics is -25.08, is the contrast between bronchitics and normals and is not significant, implying that the mean deadspace is not significantly different in bronchitics and normals.

If we wished to contrast asthmatics and bronchitics, we need to make one of them the baseline. Thus we make x_1 and x_3 the independent variables to make bronchitics the baseline and the output is shown in the second half of Table 2.7. As would be expected the Prob > F and the R^2 value are the same as the earlier

Table 2.7 Output from computer program fitting two categorical variables to deadspace from Table 2.2

Asthma and bronchitis as independent variables

Number of obs = 15, F(2,12) = 7.97, Prob > F = 0.0063
R-squared   = 0.5705 Adj R-squared = 0.4990

y	Coef.	Std. Err.	t	P>|t|	[95% Conf. Interval]	
Asthma	-44.45833	11.33229	-3.923	0.002	-69.14928	-19.76739
Bronch	-25.08333	12.78455	-1.962	0.073	-52.93848	2.771809
_cons	97.33333	9.664212	10.072	0.000	76.27683	118.3898

Asthma and Normal as independent variables

Number of obs = 15, F(2, 12) = 7.97, Prob > F = 0.0063
R-squared = 0.5705, Adj R-squared = 0.4990

y	Coef.	Std. Err.	t	P>|t|	[95% Conf. Interval]	
Asthma	-19.375	10.25044	-1.890	0.083	-41.7088	2.9588
Normal	25.08333	12.78455	1.962	0.073	-2.771809	52.93848
_cons	72.25	8.369453	8.633	0.000	54.01453	90.48547

model because these refer to the overall model which differs from the earlier one only in the formulation of the parameters. However, now the coefficients refer to the contrast with bronchitis, and we can see that the difference between asthmatics and bronchitics has a difference -19.38 with SE 10.25, which is not significant.

Thus the only significant difference is between asthmatics and normals.

This method of analysis is also known as *one-way analysis of variance*. It is a generalisation of the t-test referred to in Swinscow and Campbell.[1] One could ask what is the difference between this and simply carrying out two t-tests: asthmatics vs normals and bronchitics vs normals. In fact, the analysis of variance accomplishes two extra refinements. Firstly, the overall P-value controls for the problem of multiple testing referred to in Swinscow and Campbell.[1] By doing a number of tests against the baseline we are increasing the chances of a Type I error. The overall P-value in the F-test allows for this and since it is significant, we know that some of the contrasts must be significant. The second improvement is that in order to calculate a t-test we must find the pooled SE. In the t-test this is done from two groups, whereas in the analysis of variance it is calculated from all three, which is based on more subjects and so is more precise.

2.5 Multiple regression in action

2.5.1 Analysis of covariance

We mentioned that model (2.3) is very commonly seen in the literature. To see its application in a clinical trial consider the results of Llewellyn-Jones *et al.*,[3] part of which are given in Table 2.8. This study was a randomised-controlled trial of the effectiveness of a shared care intervention for depression in 220 subjects over the age of 65 years. Depression was measured using the Geriatric Depression Scale, taken at baseline and after 9.5 months of blinded follow-up. The figure that helps the interpretation is Figure 2.2. Here y is the depression scale after 9.5 months of treatment (continuous), x_1 is the value of the same scale at baseline and x_2 is the group variable, taking the value 1 for intervention and 0 for control.

Table 2.8 Factors affecting Geriatric Depression Scale score at follow-up

Variable	Regression coefficient (95% CI)	Standardised Regression Coefficient	P-value
Baseline score	0.73 (0.56 to 0.91)	0.56	<0.0001
Treatment Group	−1.87 (−2.97 to −0.76)	−0.22	0.0011

The *standardised regression coefficient* is not universally defined, but in this case is obtained when the *x* variable is replaced by *x* divided by its standard deviation. Thus the interpretation of the standardised regression coefficient is the amount the *y* changes for 1 standard deviation increase in *x*. One can see that the baseline values are highly correlated with the follow-up values of the score. The intervention resulted, on average, in patients with a score 1.87 units (95% CI 0.76 to 2.97) lower than those in the control group, throughout the range of the baseline values.

This analysis assumes that the treatment effect is the same for all subjects and is not related to values of their baseline scores. This possibility could be checked by the methods discussed earlier. When two groups are balanced with respect to the baseline value, one might assume that including the baseline value in the analysis will not affect the comparison of treatment groups. However, it is often worthwhile including because it can improve the precision of the estimate of the treatment effect; that is, the SEs of the treatment effects may be smaller when the baseline covariate is included.

2.5.2 Two continuous independent variables

Sorensen *et al.*[4] describe a cohort study of 4300 men, aged between 18 and 26, who had their body mass index (BMI) measured. The investigators wished to relate adult BMI to the men's birth weight and body length at birth. Potential confounding factors included gestational age, birth order, mother's marital status, age and occupation. In a multiple linear regression they found an association between birth weight (coded in units of 250 g) and BMI (allowing for confounders), regression coefficient 0.82, and SE 0.17, but not between birth length (cm) and BMI, regression coefficient 1.51, SE 3.87. Thus, for every increase in birth weight of 250 g, the BMI increases on average by 0.82 kg/m^2. The authors suggest that *in utero* factors that affect birth weight continue to have an affect even into adulthood, even allowing for factors, such as gestational age.

2.6 Assumptions underlying the models

There are a number of assumptions implicit in the choice of the model. The most fundamental assumption is that the model is *linear*. This means that each increase by one unit of an *x* variable is associated by a fixed increase in the *y* variable, irrespective of the starting value of the *x* variable.

There are a number of ways of checking this when *x* is continuous:
- For single continuous independent variables the simplest check is a visual one from a scatter plot of *y* vs *x*.

- Try transformations of the x variables ($\log x$, x^2 and $1/x$ are the commonest). There is not a simple significance test for one transformation against another, but a good guide would be if the R^2 value gets larger.
- Include a quadratic term (x^2) as well as the linear term (x) in the model. This model is the one where we fit two continuous variables, x and x^2. A significant coefficient for x^2 indicates a lack of linearity.
- Divide x into a number groups such as by quintiles. Fit separate dummy variables for the four largest quintile groups and examine the coefficients. For a linear relationship, the coefficients themselves will increase linearly.

Another fundamental assumption is that the error terms are independent of each other. An example of where this is unlikely is when the data form a time series. A simple check for sequential data for independent errors is whether the residuals are correlated, and a test known as the *Durbin–Watson* test is available in many packages. Further details are given in Chapter 6, on time series analysis. A further example of lack of independence is where the main unit of measurement is the individual, but several observations are made on each individual, and these are treated as if they came from different individuals. This is the problem of *repeated measures*. A similar type of problem occurs when groups of patients are randomised, rather than individual patients. These are discussed in Chapter 5, on repeated measures.

The model also assumes that the error terms are independent of the x variables and variance of the error term is constant (the latter goes under the more complicated term of *heteroscedascity*). A common alternative is when the error increases as one of the x variables increases, so one way of checking this assumption would be to plot the residuals, e_i, against each of the independent variables and also against the fitted values. If the model were correct one would expect to see the scatter of residuals evenly spread about the horizontal axis and not showing any pattern. A common departure from this is when the residuals fan out; that is, the scatter gets larger as the x variable gets larger. This is often also associated with nonlinearity as well, and so attempts at transforming the x variable may resolve this issue.

The final assumption is that the error term is Normally distributed. One could check this by plotting a histogram of the residuals, although the method of fitting will mean that the observed residuals e_i are likely to be closer to a Normal distribution than the true ones ε_i. The assumption of Normality is important mainly so that we can use normal theory to estimate confidence intervals (CIs) around the coefficients, but luckily with reasonably large sample sizes, the estimation method is robust to departures from Normality. Thus moderate departures from Normality are allowable. If one was concerned, then one could also use bootstrap methods and the robust standard error described in Appendix 3.

It is important to remember that the main purpose of this analysis is to assess a relationship, *not* test assumptions, so often we can come to a useful conclusion *even when the assumptions are not perfectly satisfied.*

2.7 Model sensitivity

Model sensitivity refers to how estimates are affected by subgroups of the data. Suppose we had fitted a simple regression (model (2.2)), and we were told that the estimates b_0 and b_1 altered dramatically if you delete a subset of the data, or even a single individual. This is important, because we like to think that the model applies generally, and we do not wish to find that we should have different models for different subgroups of patients.

2.7.1 Residuals, leverage and influence

There are three main issues in identifying model sensitivity to individual observations: *residuals*, *leverage* and *influence*. The residuals are the difference between the observed and fitted data: $e_i = y_i^{obs} - y_i^{fit}$. A point with a large residual is called an outlier. In general, we are interested in outliers because they may influence the estimates, but it is possible to have a large outlier which is not influential.

Another way that a point can be an outlier is if the values of the x_i are a long way from the mass of x. For a single variable, this means if x_i is a long way from $\bar{x}$. Imagine a scatter plot of y against x, with a mass of points in the bottom-left-hand corner and a single point in the top right. It is possible that this individual has unique characteristics that relate to both the x and y variables. A regression line fitted to the data will go close, or even through the isolated point. This isolated point will not have a large residual, yet if this point was deleted the regression coefficient might change dramatically. Such a point is said to have high *leverage* and this can be measured by a number, often denoted h_i; large values of h_i indicate a high leverage.

An influential point is one that has a large effect on an estimate. Effectively one fits the model with and without that point and finds the effect of the regression coefficient. One might look for points that have a large effect on b_0, or on b_1 or on other estimates such as $SE(b_1)$. The usual output is the difference in the regression coefficient for a particular variable when the point is included or excluded, scaled by the estimated SE of the coefficient. The problem is that different parameters may have different influential points. Most computer packages now produce residuals, leverages and influential points as a matter of routine. It is the task for an analyst to examine these and to identify important cases. However, just because a point is influential or has a large residual it does not follow that it should be deleted, although the data should be examined carefully for possible measurement or transcription errors. A proper analysis of such data would report such sensitivities to individual points.

2.7.2 Computer analysis: model checking and sensitivity

We will illustrate model checking and sensitivity using the deadspace, age and height data in Table 2.1.

Figure 2.1 gives us reassurance that the relationship between deadspace and height is plausibly linear. We could plot a similar graph for deadspace and age. The standard diagnostic plot is a plot of the residuals against the fitted values, and for the model fitted in Table 2.6 it is shown in Figure 2.4. There is no apparent pattern, which gives us reassurance about the error term being relatively constant and further reassurance about the linearity of the model.

The diagnostic statistics are shown in Table 2.9 where the *influence* statistics are *inf_age* associated with age and *inf_ht* associated with height. As one might expect the children with the highest leverages are the youngest (who is also the shortest) and the oldest (who is also the tallest). Note that the largest residuals are associated with small leverages. This is because points with large leverage will tend to force the line close to them.

The child with the most influence on the age coefficient is also the oldest, and removal of that child would change the standardised regression coefficient by 0.79 units. The child with the most influence on height is the shortest child.

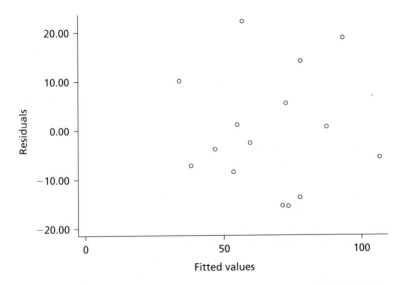

Figure 2.4 Graph of residuals against fitted values for regression model in Table 2.4 with age and height as the independent variables.

Table 2.9 Diagnostics from model fitted in Table 2.4 (output from computer program)

	Height	Age	resids	leverage	inf_age	inf_ht
1	110	5	10.06	0.33	0.22	−0.48
2	116	5	−7.19	0.23	−0.04	0.18
3	124	6	−3.89	0.15	−0.03	0.08
4	129	7	−8.47	0.15	−0.14	0.20
5	131	7	1.12	0.12	0.01	−0.02
6	138	6	22.21	0.13	−0.52	0.34
7	142	6	−2.61	0.17	0.08	−0.06
8	150	8	−15.36	0.08	0.11	−0.14
9	153	8	−15.48	0.10	0.20	−0.26
10	155	9	14.06	0.09	0.02	0.07
11	156	7	5.44	0.28	−0.24	0.25
12	159	8	−13.72	0.19	0.38	−0.46
13	164	10	0.65	0.14	0.00	0.01
14	168	11	18.78	0.19	0.29	0.08
15	174	14	−5.60	0.65	−0.79	0.42

However, neither child should be removed without strong reason. (A strong reason may be if it was discovered the child had some relevant disease, such as cystic fibrosis.)

2.8 Stepwise regression

When one has a large number of independent variables, a natural question to ask is what is the best combination of these variables to predict the y variable? To answer this, one may use *stepwise* regression that is available in a number of packages. *Step-down* or *backwards* regression starts by fitting all available variables and then discarding sequentially those that are not significant. *Step-up* or *forwards* regression starts by fitting an overall mean, and then selecting variables to add to the model according to their significance. *Stepwise* regression is a mixture of the two, where one can specify a P-value for a variable to be entered into the model, and then a P-value for a variable to be discarded. Usually one chooses a larger P-value for entry (say, 0.1) than for exclusion (say, 0.05), since variables can jointly be predictive, and separately they are not. This also favours *step-down* regression. As an example consider an outcome variable being the amount a person limps. The length of the left or right legs is not predictive, but the difference in lengths is highly predictive. Stepwise regression is best used in the *exploratory* phase of an analysis (see Chapter 1), to identify a few predictors in a mass of data, the association of which can be verified by further data collection.

There are a few problems with stepwise regression:
- The *P*-values are invalid since they do not take account of the vast number of tests that have been carried out; different methods, such as step-up and step-down, are likely to produce different models and experience shows that the same model rarely emerges when a second data set is analysed. One way of trying to counter this is to split a large data set into two, and run the stepwise procedure on both separately. Choose the variables that are common to both data sets, and fit these to the combined data set as the final model.
- Many large data sets contain missing values. With stepwise regression, usually only the subjects who have no missing values on *any* of the variables under consideration are chosen. The final model may contain only a few variables, but if one refits the model, the parameters change because now the model is being fitted to those subjects who have no missing values on only the few chosen variables, which may be a considerably larger data set than the original.
- If a categorical variable is coded as a number of dummies, some of these may be lost in the fitting process, and this changes the interpretation of the others. Thus, if we fitted x_1 and x_2 from Table 2.2, and then we lost x_2, the interpretation of x_1 is of a contrast between asthmatics with bronchitics and normals *combined*.

Thus stepwise regression is useful in the *exploratory* phase of an analysis, but not the *confirmatory* one.

2.9 Reporting the results of a multiple regression

- As a minimum, report the regression coefficients and SEs or CIs for the main independent variables, together with the adjusted R^2 for the whole model.
- If there is one main dependent variable, show a scatter plot of each independent variable vs dependent variable with the best-fit line.
- Report how the assumptions underlying the model were tested and verified. In particular is linearity plausible?
- Report any sensitivity analysis carried out.
- Report *all* the variables included in the model. For a stepwise regression, report *all* the variables that could have entered the model.
- Note that if an interaction term is included in a model, the main effects *must* be included.

2.10 Reading the results of a multiple regression

In addition to the points in Section 1.11:
- Note the value of R^2. With a large study, the coefficients in the model can be highly significant, but only explain a low proportion of the variability of the outcome variable. Thus they may be of no use for prediction.

• Are the models plausibly linear? Are there any boundaries, which may cause the slope to flatten?
• Were outliers and influential points identified, and how were they treated?
• An analysis of covariance *assumes* that the slopes are the same in each group. Is this plausible and has it been tested?

FREQUENTLY ASKED QUESTIONS

1 *Does it matter how a dummy variable is coded?*
If you have only one binary variable, then coding the dummy variable 0 and 1 is the most convenient. Coding it 1 and 2 is commonly the method in questionnaires. It will make no difference to the coefficient estimate or P-value. However it will change the value of the intercept, because now the value in the group assigned 1 will be $a + b$ and the value in the group assigned 2 will be $a + 2b$. Thus in Figure 2.2 when "asthma" is coded 0 or 1 the regression coefficient is -16.8 and the intercept is -46.3. If we had coded the variable 1 or 2 we would find the regression coefficient is still -16.8 but the intercept would be $(-46.3 - 16.8) = -63.1$. Coding the dummy variable to -1 and $+1$, (e.g. as is done in the package SAS) does not change the P-value but the coefficient is halved.

If you have a categorical variable with, say, three groups, then this will be coded with two dummy variables. As shown earlier, the overall F-statistic will be unchanged no matter which two groups are chosen to be represented by dummies, but the coefficient of group 2, say, will be dependent on whether group 1 or 3 is the omitted variable.

2 *How do I treat an ordinal independent variable?*
Most packages assume that the predictor variable, X, in a regression model is either continuous or binary. Thus one has a number of options:

(i) Treat the predictor as if it were continuous. This incorporates into the model the fact that the categories are ordered, but also assumes that equal changes in X mean equal changes in y.

(ii) Treat the predictor as if it were categorical, by fitting dummy variables to all but one of the categories. This loses the fact that the predictor is ordinal, but makes no assumption about linearity.

(iii) Dichotomise the X variable, by recoding it as binary, say 1 if X is in a particular category or above, and 0 otherwise. The cut-point should be chosen on external grounds and not because it gives the best fit to the data.

Which of these options you choose depends on a number of factors. With a large amount of data, the loss of information by ignoring the ordinality in option

(continued)

(ii) is not critical and especially if the X variable is a confounder and not of prime interest. For example, if X is age grouped in 10-year intervals, it might be better to fit dummy variables, than assume a linear relation with the y-variable.

3 *Do the assumptions underlying multiple regression matter?*

Often the assumptions underlying multiple regression are not checked, partly because the investigator is confident that they hold true and partly because mild departures are unlikely to invalidate an analysis. However, lack of independence may be obvious on empirical grounds (the data form repeated measures or a time series) and so the analysis should accommodate this from the outset. Linearity is important for inference and so may be checked by fitting transformations of the independent variables. Lack of homogeneity of variance and lack of Normality may affect the SEs and often indicate the need for a transformation of the dependent variable. The most common departure from Normality is when outliers are identified, and these should be carefully checked, particularly those with high leverage.

4 *I have a variable that I believe should be a confounder but it is not significant. Should I include it in the analysis?*

There are certain variables (such as age or sex) for which one might have strong grounds for believing that they could be confounders, but in any particular analysis might emerge as not significant. These should be retained in the analysis because, even if not significantly related to the outcome themselves, they may modify the effect of the prime independent variable.

5 *What happens if I have a dependent variable, which is 0 or 1?*

When the dependent variable is 0 or 1 then the coefficients from a linear regression are proportional to what is known as the *linear discriminant function*. This can be useful for discriminating between groups, even if the assumption about Normality of the residuals is violated. However discrimination is normally carried out now using *logistic regression* (Chapter 3).

6 *Why not analyse the difference between outcome and baseline (change score) rather than use analysis of covariance?*

Analysing change does not properly control for baseline imbalance because of what is known as regression to the mean; baseline values are negatively correlated with change and subjects with low scores at baseline will tend to increase more than those with high values. However, if the correlation between baseline and follow-up measurements is large (say, $r > 0.8$) and randomisation has ensured that baseline values are comparable between groups, then an analysis of change scores may produce lower SEs. Note that if the change score is the dependent variable and baseline is included as an independent variable, then the results will be the same as an analysis of covariance.

EXERCISE

Melchart et al.[5] describe a randomised trial of acupuncture in patients with tension-type headache with 2:1 randomisation to either acupuncture for 8 weeks or a waiting list control. Partial results are given in the following table.

Results from Melchart et al.[5]

	Acupuncture	Waiting list
Baseline	17.5 (6.9) ($n = 132$)	17.3 (6.9) ($n = 75$)
After treatment	9.9 (8.7) ($n = 118$)	16.3 (7.4) ($n = 63$)

Values are represented as days with headache during a 28-day period (Mean (SD)).

Difference between groups after treatment: 5.7 days (95% CI 4.2 to 7.2) $P < 0.001$.

Analysis of covariance adjusting for baseline value – Difference between groups after treatment: 5.8 days (95% CI 4.0 to 7.6) $P < 0.001$.

1 Give three assumptions made for the analysis of covariance.
2 What evidence do we have that these may not be satisfied?
3 Contrast the two CIs.
4 What other data might one like to see?

References

1. Swinscow TDV, Campbell MJ. *Statistics at Square One*, 10th edn. London: BMJ Books, 2002.
2. Draper NR, Smith H. *Applied Regression Analysis*, 3rd edn. New York: John Wiley, 1998.
3. Llewellyn-Jones RH, Baikie KA, Smithers H, Cohen J, Snowdon J, Tennant CC. Multifaceted shared care intervention for late life depression in residential care: randomised controlled trial. *Br Med J* 1999; **319:** 676–82.
4. Sorensen HT, Sabroe S, Rothman KJ, Gillman M, Fischer P, Sorensen TIA. Relation between weight and length at birth and body mass index in young adulthood: cohort study. *Br Med J* 1997; **315:** 1137.
5. Melchart D, Streng A, Hoppe A, Brinkhaus B, Witt C, *et al.* Acupuncture in patients with tension-type headache: randomised controlled trial. *Br Med J* 2005; **331:** 376–82.

Chapter 3 **Logistic regression**

Summary

The Chi-squared test is used for testing the association between two binary variables.[1] Logistic regression is a generalisation of the Chi-squared test to examine the association of a binary dependent variable with one or more independent variables that can be binary, categorical (more than two categories) or continuous. Logistic regression is also useful for analysing *case–control* studies. Matched case–control studies require a particular analysis known as *conditional logistic regression*.

3.1 The model

The dependent variable can be described as an *event* which is either present or absent (sometimes termed "success" or "failure"). Thus, an event might be the presence of a disease in a survey or cure from disease in a clinical trial. We wish to examine factors associated with the event. Since we can rarely predict exactly whether an event will happen or not, what we in fact look for are factors associated with the *probability* of an event happening.

There are two situations to be considered:

1 When all the independent variables are categorical, and so one can form tables in which each cell has individuals with the same values of the independent variables. As a consequence one can calculate the proportion of subjects for whom an event happens. For example, one might wish to examine the presence or absence of a disease by gender (two categories) and social class (five categories). Thus, one could form a table with the 10 social class-by-gender categories and examine the proportion of subjects with disease in each grouping.

2 When the data table contains as many cells as there are individuals and the observed proportions of subjects with disease in each cell must be 0 out of 1 or 1 out of 1.

This can occur when at least one of the independent variables is continuous, but of course can also be simply a consequence of the way the data are input. It is possible that each individual has a unique set of predictors and we may not wish to group them.

If the data are in the form of tables most computer packages will provide a separate set of commands to carry out an analysis. Preserving the individual cases leads to the same regression estimates and allows a more flexible analysis. This is discussed further in Section 3.3.

The purpose of statistical analysis is to take *samples* to estimate *population parameters*.[1] In logistic regression we model the population parameters. If we consider the categorical-grouped case first, denote the population probability of an event for a cell i by π_i. This is also called the "expected" value. Thus, for an unbiased coin the population or expected probability for a "head" is 0.5. The dependent variable, y_i, is the observed proportion of events in the cell (say, the proportion of heads in a set of tosses) and we write $E(y_i) = \pi_i$ where E denotes "expected value". Also recall that if an event has probability π_i, then the *odds* for that event are $\pi_i/(1 - \pi_i)$ to 1. Thus, the *odds* of a head to a tail are 1 to 1.

The model is

$$\log_e \frac{\pi_i}{1 - \pi_i} = \text{logit}(\pi_i) = \beta_0 + \beta_1 X_{i1} + \cdots + \beta_p X_{ip}, \qquad (3.1)$$

where the independent variables are $X_{i1}, \ldots, X_{ip}$.

The term on the left-hand side of the equation is the log odds of success, and is often called the *logistic* or *logit* transform.

The reason why model (3.1) is useful is that the coefficients, β, are related to the *odds ratio* (OR) in 2 × 2 tables. Suppose we had only one covariate X, which was binary and simply takes the values 0 or 1. Then the OR associated with X and the outcome is given by $\exp(\beta)$ (note *not* the "relative risk" as is sometimes stated). If X is continuous, then $\exp(\beta)$ is the OR of an event associated with a unit increase in X.

The main justification for the logit transformation is that the OR is a natural parameter to use for binary outcomes, and the logit transformation relates this to the independent variables in a convenient manner. It can also be justified as follows. The right-hand side of equation (3.1) is potentially unbounded; that is, can range from minus to plus infinity. On the left-hand side, a probability must lie between 0 and 1. An OR must lie between 0 and infinity. A log OR, or logit, is unbounded and has the same potential range as the right-hand side of equation (3.1).

Note that at this stage, the *observed* values of the dependent variable are not in the equation. They are linked to the model by the Binomial distribution (described in Appendix 2). Thus, in cell i if we observe y_i successes in n_i subjects, we assume that the y_i are distributed Binomially with probability π_i. The parameters in the model are estimated by maximum likelihood (also discussed in Appendix 2). Of course, we do not know the population values π_i, and in the modelling process we substitute into the model the estimated or fitted values.

Often, by analogy to multiple regression, the model is described in the literature as above, but with the observed proportion, $p_i = y_i/n_i$, replacing π_i. This misses out on the second part of a model, the error distribution, that links the two. One could, in fact, use the observed proportions and fit the model by least squares as in multiple regression. In the cases where the p_is are not close to 0 or 1, this will often do well – although the interpretation of the model is different from that of equation (3.1) – as the link with ORs is missing. With modern computers the method of maximum likelihood is easy and is also to be preferred. When the dependent variable is 0/1, the logit of the dependent variable does not exist. This may lead some people to believe that logistic regression is impossible in these circumstances. However, as explained earlier the model uses the logit of the *expected* value, not the observed value, and the model ensures that the expected value is >0 and <1.

We may wish to calculate the probability of an event. Suppose we have estimated the coefficients in (3.1) to be $b_0, b_1, \ldots, b_p$. As in Chapter 1 we write the estimated linear predictor as

$$LP_i = b_0 + b_1 X_{i1} + \cdots + b_p X_{ip}.$$

Then equation (3.1) can be written as

$$\hat{\pi}_i = \frac{e^{LP_i}}{1 + e^{LP_i}} \tag{3.2}$$

where $\hat{\pi}_i$ is an estimate of π_i and estimates the probability of an event from the model. These are the predicted or fitted values for y_i. A good model will give predictions $\hat{\pi}_i$ close to the observed proportions y_i/n_i.

Further details of logistic regression are given in Collett[2] and Hosmer and Lemeshow.[3]

3.2 Uses of logistic regression

1 As a substitute for multiple regression, when the outcome variable is binary in cross-sectional and cohort studies and in clinical trials. Thus, we would use logistic regression to investigate the relationship between a causal variable and a binary output variable, allowing for confounding variables which can be categorical or continuous.

2 As a discriminant analysis, to try and find factors that discriminate two groups. Here the outcome would be a binary variable indicating membership to a group. For example one might want to discriminate men and women on psychological test results.

3 To develop prognostic indicators, such as the risk of complications from surgery.

4 To analyse case–control studies and matched case–control studies.

3.3 Interpreting a computer output: grouped analysis

Most computer packages have different procedures for the situations when the data appear in a grouped table, and when they refer to individuals. It is usually easier to store data on an individual basis, since it can be used for a variety of purposes. However, the coefficients and standard errors (SEs) of a logistic regression analysis will be exactly the same for the grouped procedure when the independent variables are all categorical, and where the dependent variable is the number of successes in the group and for the ungrouped procedure where the dependent variable is simply 0/1. In general, it is easier to examine the goodness-of-fit of the model in the grouped case.

3.3.1 One binary independent variable

Consider the example given in Swinscow and Campbell[1] in which the association between breast and bottle feeding at 3 months was examined for printers' and farmers' wives.

We can define an event as a baby being breastfed for <3 months and we have a single categorical variable X_1 which takes the value 1 if the mother were a printer's wife and 0 if she were a farmer's wife. The data are given in Table 3.1.

Table 3.1 Numbers of wives of printers and farmers who breastfed their babies for less than 3 months or for 3 months or more

	<3 months	$\geqslant 3$ months	Total
Printers' wives	36	14	50
Farmers' wives	30	25	55
Total	66	39	105

From Swinscow and Campbell[1] (Table 8.3).

We can rewrite Table 3.1 for the computer either as for a grouped analysis

y	n	Occupation (1 = printer, 0 = farmer)
36	50	1
30	55	0

or as the following 105 rows for an ungrouped analysis

Row number	y (breastfeeding) 1 for <3 months, 0 for ≥3 months		Occupation (1 = printer, 0 = farmer)
1	1		1
		(36 times)	
37	1		0
		(30 times)	
67	0		1
		(14 times)	
81	0		0
		(25 times)	

It is simple to show that the relative risk of breastfeeding for <3 months is $(36/50)/(30/55) = 1.32$ for printers' wives relative to farmers' wives and the OR is $(36/14)/(30/25) = 2.14$. The reason for the discrepancy is that when the outcome, in this case breastfeeding, is common the relative risks and ORs tend to differ. When the outcome is rare (e.g. probability of an event <0.1) then the OR and relative risk will be closer. For a discussion of the relative merits of ORs and relative risk see Swinscow and Campbell.[1] In Chapter 6, we will show how to obtain the relative risk directly.

The output for a logistic regression for these data (in the second form) is shown in Table 3.2. The first section of the Table gives the fit for a constant term and the second the fit of the term occupation. The model for the first section is

$$\log_e \frac{\pi_i}{1 - \pi_i} = \beta_0$$

and for the second

$$\log_e \frac{\pi_i}{1 - \pi_i} = \beta_0 + \beta_1 \times \text{Occupation}.$$

Table 3.2 Output from a logistic regression program using data in Table 3.1

```
Logit estimates                        Number of obs   =       105
                                       LR chi2(0)      =      0.00
                                       Prob > chi2     =        .
Log likelihood = -69.26972             Pseudo R2       =    0.0000
---------------------------------------------------------------------
_outcome |    Coef.   Std. Err.    z    P>|z|  [95% Conf. Interval]
---------+-----------------------------------------------------------
   _cons | .5260931   .2019716   2.60   0.009   .130236     .9219502
---------------------------------------------------------------------

Logit estimates                        Number of obs   =       105
                                       LR chi2(1)      =      3.45
                                       Prob > chi2     =    0.0631
Log likelihood = -67.543174            Pseudo R2       =    0.0249
---------------------------------------------------------------------
_outcome |    Coef.   Std. Err.    z    P>|z|  [95% Conf. Interval]
---------+-----------------------------------------------------------
 occuptn | .7621401   .415379    1.83   0.067  -.0519878    1.576268
   _cons | .1823216   .2708013   0.67   0.501  -.3484392    .7130823
---------------------------------------------------------------------

Logit estimates                        Number of obs   =       105
                                       LR chi2(1)      =      3.45
                                       Prob > chi2     =    0.0631
Log likelihood = -67.543174            Pseudo R2       =    0.0249
---------------------------------------------------------------------
_outcome |    Odds   Std. Err.    z    P>|z|  [95% Conf. Interval]
         |   Ratio
---------+-----------------------------------------------------------
 occuptn |2.142857   .8900978   1.83   0.067   .9493405    4.83687
---------------------------------------------------------------------
```

The output can be requested in terms of either the coefficients in the model or the ORs, and here we give both. The output also gives the log-likelihood values, which are derived in Appendix 2, and can be thought of as a sort of residual sum of squares.

The log-likelihood for the model without the occupation term is $L_0 = -69.27$ and with the occupation term is $L_1 = -67.54$. The difference multiplied by -2 is the "LR chi2(1)" term (LR for likelihood ratio), which is 3.45. This can be interpreted as a Chi-squared statistic with 1 degree of freedom (d.f.). This is further described in Appendix 2. It can be seen that the LR Chi-squared statistic for this model has 1 d.f., since it has only one term (occupation), and is not significant ($P = 0.0631$).

The "Pseudo R2" is given by $1 - L_1/L_0$. It is analogous to the R^2 term in linear regression which gives the proportion of variance accounted for by the model. This is less easy to interpret in the binary case, and it is suggested that one considers only the rough magnitude of the Pseudo R2. In this case, a value of 0.0249 implies that the model does not fit particularly well since only a small proportion of the variance is accounted for.

The Wald statistic, which is the ratio of the estimate b to its SE, that is, $z = b/SE(b) = (0.7621/0.4154) = 1.83$. The square of this, 3.3489, is close to the LR statistic, and the corresponding P-value (0.067) is close to the LR Chi-squared value of 0.0631.

The conventional Chi-squared statistic, described in Swinscow and Campbell,[1] is neither the Wald nor the LR and is in fact the third of the statistics derived from likelihood theory, the score statistic (see Appendix 2). This has value 3.418, and is very close to the other two statistics.

If b_1 is the estimate of β_1 then $\exp(b_1)$ is the estimated OR associated with X_1. The coefficient in the model is 0.7621, and the OR is given by $\exp(0.7621) = 2.143$. Thus, the ORs of printers' wives breastfeeding for <3 months are more than twice that of farmer's wives.

A 95% confidence interval (CI) for β (which is a log odds) is given by $b \pm 1.96 \times SE(b)$. This is sometimes known as a *Wald confidence interval* (see Section 3.4) since it is based on the Wald test. Thus, a 95% CI for the OR is $\exp\{b - 1.96 \times SE(b)\}$ to $\exp\{b + 1.96 \times SE(b)\}$. This is asymmetric about OR, in contrast to the CIs in linear regression. For example, from Table 3.2, the CI for the estimate is $\exp(0.7621 - 1.96 \times 0.4154)$ to $\exp(0.7621 + 1.96 \times 0.4154)$ or 0.949 to 4.837, which is asymmetric about 2.143. Note that the CI includes 1, which is to be expected since the significance test is non-significant at $P = 0.05$. In general, this will hold true, but there can be slight discrepancies with the significance test especially if the OR is large because the test of significance may be based on the LR test or the score test, whereas the CI is usually based on the Wald test.

3.3.2 Two binary independent variables
Consider the data supplied by Julious and Mullee[4] on mortality of diabetics in a cohort study given in Table 3.3.

Table 3.3 Data from Julious and Mullee[4] on mortality of diabetics

		Died	Total	%
Age <40	Non-insulin dependent	0	15	0
	Insulin dependent	1	130	0.1
Age $\geqslant 40$	Non-insulin dependent	218	529	41.2
	Insulin dependent	104	228	45.6
All ages	Non-insulin dependent	218	544	40.1
	Insulin dependent	105	358	29.3

Note that over all ages a greater percentage of deaths occur in the non-insulin group, but when we split by age a greater proportion of deaths occurs in each of the insulin-dependent groups. This is an example of *Simpson's Paradox*. The explanation is that age is a confounding factor, since non-insulin-dependent diabetes is predominantly a disease of older age, and of course old people are more likely to die than young people. In this case the confounding is so strong it reverses the apparent association.

To analyse this we code the data for a grouped analysis as follows:

Dead	Total	Group Dependence = 1 Non-dependence = 0	Age <40 = 0 ⩾40 = 1
0	15	0	0
1	130	1	0
218	529	0	1
104	228	1	1

The output from a logistic regression using data in Table 3.3 is given in Table 3.4. In the first part of the analysis the OR associated with group is 0.62, suggesting that insulin dependence (when group = 1) has a lower risk than non-dependence. When age is included as a factor, this changes to an OR of 1.2,

Table 3.4 Output from a logistic regression using data in Table 3.3

```
Logit estimates                          Number of obs  =      902
                                         LR chi2(1)     =    10.98
                                         Prob > chi2    =   0.0009
Log likelihood = -582.89735              Pseudo R2      =   0.0093
------------------------------------------------------------------
_outcome |    Odds   Std. Err.    z    P>|z|   [95% Conf. Interval]
         |    Ratio
---------+--------------------------------------------------------
   Group | .6206259  .0902169  -3.28   0.001   .466762     .8252096
------------------------------------------------------------------

Logit estimates                          Number of obs  =      902
                                         LR chi2(2)     =   133.63
                                         Prob > chi2    =   0.0000
Log likelihood = -521.57263              Pseudo R2      =   0.1136
------------------------------------------------------------------
_outcome |    Odds   Std. Err.    z    P>|z|   [95% Conf. Interval]
         |    Ratio
---------+--------------------------------------------------------
   Group | 1.19919    .19123   1.14   0.255   .8773042    1.639176
     age | 118.8813  120.1647   4.73   0.000   16.39542    861.9942
------------------------------------------------------------------
```

which is >1 and suggests that an adverse effect of insulin dependence albeit non-statistically significant. It should be stressed that this no way proves that starting to take insulin for diabetes *causes* a higher mortality; other confounding factors, as yet unmeasured, may also be important.

It should be stressed that this procedure is the logistic equivalence to ANCOVA described in Section 2.5.1. Here the covariate, age, is binary, but it could be included as a continuous covariate and Julious and Mullee[4] show that including age as a continuous variable changes the relative risk from 0.69 to 1.15, which is similar to the changes in the ORs observed here.

As usual one has to be aware of assumptions. The main one here is that the OR for insulin dependence is the same in the younger and older groups. There are not enough data to test that here. Another assumption is that the cut-off point at age 40 years was chosen on clinical grounds and not by looking at the data to file the best possible result for the investigator. One would need some reassurance of this in the text!

3.4 Logistic regression in action

Lavie *et al.*[5] surveyed 2677 adults referred to a sleep clinic with suspected sleep apnoea (when a sleeper temporarily stops breathing). They developed an apnoea severity index, and related this to the presence or absence of hypertension.

They wished to answer two questions:

1 Is the apnoea index predictive of hypertension, allowing for age, sex and body mass index (BMI)?
2 Is sex a predictor of hypertension, allowing for the other covariates?

The results are given in Table 3.5 and the authors chose to give the regression coefficients (log odds) and the Wald confidence interval.

The coefficient associated with the dummy variable sex is 0.161, so the odds of having hypertension for a man are $\exp(0.161) = 1.17$ times that of a woman in this study. On the OR scale the 95% CI is $\exp(-0.061)$ to $\exp(0.383) = 0.94$ to 1.47. Note that this includes 1 (as we would expect

Table 3.5 Risk factors for hypertension[5]

Risk factor	Estimate (log odds)	(Wald 95% CI)	OR
Age (10 years)	0.805	(0.718 to 0.892)	2.24
Sex (male)	0.161	(−0.061 to 0.383)	1.17
BMI (5 kg/m^2)	0.332	(0.256 to 0.409)	1.39
Apnoea index (10 units)	0.116	(0.075 to 0.156)	1.12

since the CI for the regression coefficient includes 0) and so we cannot say that sex is a significant predictor of hypertension in this study. We interpret the age coefficient by saying that, if we had two people of the same sex, and given that their BMI and apnoea index were also the same, but one subject was 10 years elder than the other, then we would predict that the older subject would be 2.24 times more likely to have hypertension. The reason for the choice of 10 years is because that is how age was scaled. Note that factors that are additive on the log scale are multiplicative on the odds scale. Thus a man who is 10 years older than a woman is predicted to be $2.24 \times 1.17 = 2.62$ times more likely to have hypertension. Thus the model assumes that age and sex act independently on hypertension, and so the risks multiply. This can be checked by including an interaction term between age and sex in the model as described in Chapter 2. If this is found to be significant, it implies that there is *effect modification* between age and sex, and hence if the interaction was positive it would imply that an older man is at much greater risk of hypertension than would be predicted by his age and sex separately.

3.5 Model checking

There are a number of ways the model may fail to describe the data well. Some of these are the same as those discussed in Section 2.7 for linear regression, such as linearity of the coefficients in the linear predictor, influential observations and lack of an important confounder. It is important to look for observations whose removal has a large influence on the model coefficients. These *influential points* are handled in logistic regression in a similar way to that described for multiple regression in Chapter 2, and some computer packages give measures of influence of individual points in logistic regression. These can be checked, and the model refitted omitting them, to see how stable the model is.

Defining residuals and outlying observations is more difficult in logistic regression, when the outcome is 0 or 1, and some parts of model checking are different to the linear regression situation. Further details are given by Collett[2] and Campbell.[6]

Issues particularly pertinent to logistic regression are: lack of fit, "extra-Binomial" variation, the logistic transform.

3.5.1 Lack of fit

If the independent variables are all categorical, then one can compare the observed proportions in each of the cells and those predicted by the model. However, if some of the input variables are continuous, one has to group the predicted values in some way. Hosmer and Lemeshow[3] suggest a number of methods. One suggestion is to group the predicted probabilities from the model $\hat{\pi}_i$ and $1 - \hat{\pi}_i$ into tenths (by deciles), and compute the predicted number of successes between each decile as the sum of the predicted probabilities for those individuals in that group. Fewer groups may be used if the number of observations is small. The observed number of successes and failures can be compared using a Chi-squared distribution with 8 d.f. The reason for there being 8 d.f. is that the basic table has 10 rows and 2 columns (either predicted success or predicted failure) and so 20 initial units. The proportion in each row must add to 1, which gives 10 constraints and the proportion in each column is fixed, to give another 2 constraints and so the number of d.f. is $20 - 10 - 2 = 8$. A well fitting model should be able to predict the observed successes and failures in each group with some accuracy. A significant Chi-squared value indicates that the model is a poor description of the data.

3.5.2 "Extra-Binomial" variation

Unlike multiple regression, where the size of the residual variance is not specified in advance and is estimated from the data, in logistic regression a consequence of the Binomial model is that the residual variance is predetermined. However, the value specified by the model may be less (and sometimes greater) than that observed, and this is known as extra-Binomial variation. When the variance is greater than expected, then it is known as "over-dispersion" and it can occur when the data are not strictly independent. For example, repeated outcomes within an individual, or patients grouped by general practitioner. While the estimate of the regression coefficients is not unduly affected, the estimates of the SEs are usually underestimated, leading to CIs that are too narrow. In the past, this has been dealt with by an approximate method; for example, by scaling the SEs upwards to allow for the underestimation, but not changing the estimates of the coefficients. However, this situation is now viewed as a special case of what is known as a *random effects* model in which one (or more) of the regression coefficients β is regarded as random with a mean and variance that can be estimated, rather than fixed. This will be described in Chapter 5.

3.5.3 The logistic transform is inappropriate

The logistic transform is not the only one that converts a probability ranging from 0 to 1 to a variable that, potentially, can range from minus infinity to plus infinity. Other examples are the *probit* and the *complementary log–log* transform given by $\log[-\log(1 - \pi)]$. The latter is useful when the events (such as deaths) occur during a cohort study and leads to survival analyses (see Chapter 4). Some packages enable one to use different link functions and usually they will give similar results. The logistic link is the easiest to interpret and the one generally recommended.

3.6 Interpreting computer output: ungrouped analysis

A consecutive series of 170 patients were scored for risk of complications following abdominal operations with an APACHE risk score (a scoring system based on clinical signs and symptoms), which in this study ranged from 0 to 27 (Johnson et al.[7]). The patients' weights (in kg) were also measured. The outcome was whether the complications after the operation were mild or severe. Here both input variables are continuous. The output is given in Table 3.6. Here the coefficients are expressed as ORs. The interpretation of the model is that, *for a fixed weight*, a subject who scores one unit higher on the APACHE will have an increased OR of severe complications of 1.9 and this is highly significant ($P < 0.001$).

As an illustration of whether the model is a good fit, we see the Hosmer–Lemeshow statistic discussed above is not significant (since the d.f. exceeds the statistic we do not need tables to decide this) indicating that the observed counts and those predicted by the model are quite close, and thus the model describes the data reasonably well. In practice, investigators use the Hosmer–Lemeshow statistic to reassure themselves that the model describes the data and so they can interpret the coefficients. However, one can object to the idea of using a significance test to determine goodness-of-fit, before using another test to determine whether coefficients are significant. If the first test is not significant, it does not tell us that the model is true, but only that we do not have enough evidence to reject it. Since no model is exactly true, with enough data the goodness-of-fit test will always reject the model. However, the model

Table 3.6 Output from a logistic regression on data from abdominal operations[7]

```
Logit estimates                    Number of obs   =      170
                                   LR chi2(2)      =   107.01
                                   Prob > chi2     =   0.0000
Log likelihood = -56.866612        Pseudo R2       =   0.4848
- - - - - - - - - - - - - - - - - - - - - - - - - - - - - - - - - -
severity |     Odds  Std. Err.     z   P>|z|  [95% Conf. Interval]
         |    Ratio
- - - - -+- - - - - - - - - - - - - - - - - - - - - - - - - - - - -
  apache | 1.898479  .2008133   6.060  0.000   1.543012    2.335836
  weight | 1.039551  .0148739   2.711  0.007   1.010804    1.069116
- - - - - - - - - - - - - - - - - - - - - - - - - - - - - - - - - -
Logistic model for severity, goodness-of-fit test
(Table collapsed on quantiles of estimated probabilities)

     number of observations  = 170
          number of groups   =  10
   Hosmer-Lemeshow chi2(8)   =   4.94

   Prob > chi2 = 0.7639
```

may be "good enough" for a valid analysis. If the model does not fit, is it valid to make inferences from the model? In general, the answer is "yes", but care is needed!

A further check on the model is to look at the influential points and these are available in many packages now. In STATA an overall influential statistic, labelled dfbeta is available, but not influential statistics for each of the regression parameters separately as in multiple regression. Table 3.7 gives the output when the most influential point has been removed, and we can be reassured that the inference is not changed. Other investigations might be to examine the sensitivity and specificity of the linear combination of APACHE score and weight to decide on an optimum cut-off for prediction.

3.6.1 Logit/logistic/log-linear

Readers of computer manuals may come across a different form of model known as a *log-linear* model. Log-linear models are used to analyse large contingency tables and can be used to analyse binary data instead of logistic regression. Some earlier computer programs only allowed log-linear models. However, in general they are more difficult to interpret than logistic regression models. They differ from logistic models in that:

- There is no clear division between dependent and independent variables.
- In logistic regression the independent variables can be continuous, in log-linear models they must be categorical.
- In log-linear models one has to include all the variables, dependent and independent, into the model first. An association between a dependent and independent variable is measured by fitting an interaction term. Thus for a log-linear model, in the Lavie *et al.*[5] study example, one would first have to split age into groups, say "young" and "old" (since age is continuous). One would then have to fit parameters corresponding to the proportion

Table 3.7 Output from a logistic regression on data from abdominal operations with the most influential observation removed[7]

```
                                    Number of obs   =        169
                                    LR chi2(2)      =     111.95
                                    Prob > chi2     =     0.0000
Log likelihood = −53.962693         Pseudo R2       =     0.5091
------------------------------------------------------------------
severity |    Odds   Std. Err.    z    P>|z|   [95% Conf. Interval]
         |    Ratio
---------+--------------------------------------------------------
  apache | 2.001762  .2316818   6.00   0.000   1.595494     2.51148
  weight | 1.04362   .015606    2.86   0.004   1.013477     1.07466
------------------------------------------------------------------
```

of subjects with and without hypertension and who are in the old or young age group before fitting a parameter corresponding to the interaction between the two to assess whether age and hypertension were associated. By contrast, in logistic regression, the presence or absence of hypertension is unequivocally the dependent variable and age an independent variable.

3.7 Case–control studies

One of the main uses of logistic regression is in the analysis of case–control studies. It is a happy fact that an OR is reversible.[1] Thus, the OR is the same whether we consider the odds of printers' wives being more likely to breastfeed for >3 months than farmers' wives, or the odds of those who breastfeed for >3 months being more likely to be printers' wives than farmers' wives. This reversal of logic occurs in case–control studies, where we select cases with a disease and controls without the disease. We then investigate the amount of exposure to a suspected cause that each has had. This is in contrast to a cohort study, where we consider those exposed or not exposed to a suspected cause, and then follow them up for disease development.

If we employ logistic regression, and code the dependent variable as 1 if the subject is a case and 0 if is a control, then the estimates of the coefficients associated with exposure are the log ORs, which, provided the disease is relatively rare, will provide valid estimates of the relative risk for the exposure variable.

3.8 Interpreting computer output: unmatched case–control study

Consider the meta-analysis of four case–control studies described in Altman et al.[8] from Wald et al. (Table 3.8).[9]

Table 3.8 Exposure to passive smoking among female lung cancer cases and controls in four studies[9]

Study	Lung cancer cases		Controls		OR
	Exposed	Unexposed	Exposed	Unexposed	
1	14	8	61	72	2.07
2	33	8	164	32	0.80
3	13	11	15	10	0.79
4	91	43	254	148	1.23

For the computer Table 3.8 is rewritten as:

Y (cases)	n (cases + controls)	Exposed	Study
14	75	1	1
8	80	0	1
33	197	1	2
etc.			

In the above table there are eight rows, being the number of unique study × exposure combinations. The dependent variable for the model is the number of cases. One also has to specify the total number of cases and controls for each row. The output from a logistic regression program is given in Table 3.9. Here *study* is a four-level categorical variable, which is a confounder and modelled with three dummy variables as described in Chapter 2. This is known as a *fixed-effects* analysis. Chapter 5 gives a further discussion on the use of dummy variables in cases such as these. The program gives the option of getting the output as the log odds (the regression coefficients) or the OR. The main result is that lung cancer and passive smoking are

Table 3.9 Output from a logistic regression program for the case–control study in Table 3.3

```
Logit estimates                      Number of obs   =      977
                                     LR chi2(4)      =    30.15
                                     Prob > chi2     =   0.0000
Log likelihood = -507.27463          Pseudo R2       =   0.0289
```

_outcome	Coef.	Std. Err.	z	P>|z|	[95% Conf. Interval]	
Istudy_2	.1735811	.292785	0.593	0.553	-.4002669	.7474292
Istudy_3	1.74551	.3673518	4.752	0.000	1.025514	2.465506
Istudy_4	.6729274	.252246	2.668	0.008	.1785343	1.16732
exposed	.1802584	.1703595	1.058	0.290	-.1536401	.5141569
_cons	-1.889435	.2464887	-7.665	0.000	-2.372544	-1.406326

_outcome	Odds Ratio	Std. Err.	z	P>|z|	[95% Conf. Interval]	
Istudy_2	1.189557	.3482845	0.593	0.553	.6701412	2.111565
Istudy_3	5.728823	2.104494	4.752	0.000	2.788528	11.76944
Istudy_4	1.959967	.4943937	2.668	0.008	1.195464	3.213371
exposed	1.197527	.2040101	1.058	0.290	.8575806	1.672228

associated with an OR of 1.198, with 95% CI 0.858 to 1.672. The Pseudo R2 which is automatically given by STATA is difficult to interpret and should not be quoted. It is printed automatically and illustrates one of the hazards of reading routine output.

3.9 Matched case–control studies

In matched case–control studies each case is matched directly with one or more controls. For a valid analysis the matching should be taken into account. An obvious method would be to fit dummy variables as strata for each of the matched groups. However, it can be shown that this will produce biased estimates.[10] Instead we use a method known as *conditional logistic regression*. In a simple 2 × 2 table this gives a result equivalent to a McNemar's test.[1] It is a flexible method, that with most modern softwares allow cases to have differing numbers of controls; it is not required to have exact 1:1 matching.

The logic for a *conditional* likelihood is quite complex, but the argument can be simplified. Suppose in a matched case–control study with exactly one control per case we had a logistic model such as equation (3.1), and for pair i the probability of an event for the case was π_{i0} and for the control π_{i1}. Given that we know that one of the pair *must* be the case, that is, there must be one and only one event in the pair, *conditional* on the pair, the probability of the event happening for the case is simply $\pi_{i0}/(\pi_{i0} + \pi_{i1})$. As an example suppose you knew that a husband and wife team had won the lottery, and the husband had bought 5 tickets and the wife 1. Then if you were asked the probability that the husband had won the lottery (knowing that either he or his wife had won), he would be 5 times more likely than his wife, that is, a conditional probability of 5/6 relative to 1/6. We can form a conditional likelihood by multiplying the probabilities for each case–control pair, and maximise it in a manner similar to that for ordinary logistic regression and now this is simply achieved with many computer packages.

The model is the same as equation (3.1), but the method of estimating the parameters is different, using conditional likelihood rather than unconditional likelihood. Any factor which is the same in the case–control set, for example a matching factor, cannot appear as an independent variable in the model.[1]

3.10 Interpreting computer output: matched case–control study

These data are taken from Eason *et al.*[11] and described in Altman *et al.*[8] Thirty-five patients who died in hospital from asthma were individually matched for sex and age with 35 control subjects who had been discharged

Table 3.10 Adequacy of monitoring in hospital of 35 deaths and matched survivors with asthma[11]

		Deaths (cases)	
		Monitoring	
		Inadequate	Adequate
Survivors (controls)	Inadequate	10	3
	Adequate	13	9

Table 3.11 Data from Table 3.3 written for a computer analysis using conditional logistic regression

Pair number	Case–control (1 = death, 0 = survival)	Monitoring (1 = inadequate, 0 = adequate)
1	1	1
1	0	1
	(for 10 pairs)	
11	1	1
11	0	0
	(for 13 pairs)	
24	1	0
24	0	1
	(for 3 pairs)	
27	1	0
27	0	0
	(for 9 pairs)	

from the same hospital in the preceding year. The adequacy of monitoring of the patients was independently assessed and the results are given in Table 3.10.

For a computer analysis this may be written as a datafile with $35 \times 2 = 70$ rows, one for each case and control as shown in Table 3.11. For example, the first block refers to the 10 deaths and 10 survivors for whom monitoring is inadequate.

The logic for conditional logistic regression is the same as for McNemar's test. When the monitoring is the same for both case and control, the pair do not contribute to the estimate of the OR. It is only when they differ that we can calculate an OR.

From Table 3.10, the estimated OR of dying in hospital associated with inadequate monitoring is given by the ratio of the numbers of the two discordant pairs, namely $13/3 = 4.33$.

Table 3.12 Output from conditional logistic regression of the matched case–control study in Table 3.8

```
Conditional (fixed-effects) logistic    Number of obs   =       70
                            regression  LR chi2(1)      =     6.74
                                        Prob > chi2     =   0.0094
Log likelihood = -20.891037             Pseudo R2       =   0.1389

----------------------------------------------------------------
 deaths |      Odds   Std. Err.     z    P>|z|   [95% Conf. Interval]
        |     Ratio
--------|-------------------------------------------------------
monitor | 4.333333   2.775524   2.289   0.022   1.234874   15.20623
----------------------------------------------------------------
```

The results of the conditional logistic regression are given in Table 3.12.

The *P*-value for the Wald test is 0.022, which is significant, suggesting that inadequate monitoring increases the risk of death. The *P*-value for the LR is 0.0094. Note the disparity between the LR test and the Wald test *P*-values. This is because the numbers in the table are small and the distribution discrete and so the approximations that all the methods use are less accurate. The McNemar's Chi-square (a score test) is $(13 - 3)^2/(13 + 3) = 6.25$ with $P = 0.012$, which is mid-way between the LR and the Wald test. Each value can be regarded as valid, and in cases of differences it is important to state which test was used for obtaining the *P*-value and perhaps quote more than one test. This is in contrast to linear regression in Chapter 2, where the three methods will all coincide.

The OR is estimated as 4.33 with 95% CI 1.23 to 15.21. This CI differs somewhat from the CI given in Altman *et al.*,[8] because an exact method was used there, which is preferable with small numbers.

Note that the advantage of conditional logistic regression over a simple McNemar's test is that other covariates could be easily incorporated into the model. In the above example, we might also have measured the use of bronchodilators for all 70 subjects, as a risk factor for dying in hospital.

3.11 Conditional logistic regression in action

Churchill *et al.*[12] used a matched case–control study in which the cases were teenagers who had become pregnant over a 3-year period. Three age-matched controls, closest in age to the case, who had no recorded teenage pregnancy were identified from within the same practice. The results were analysed by conditional logistic regression and showed that cases were more likely to have consulted a doctor in the year before conception than controls (OR: 2.70, 95% CI 1.56 to 4.66).

3.12 Reporting the results of logistic regression

- Summarise the logistic regression to include the number of observations in the analysis, the coefficient of the explanatory variable with its SE and/or the OR and the 95% CI for the OR and the *P*-value.
- If a predictor variable is continuous, then it is often helpful to scale it to ease interpretation. For example, it is easier to think of the increased risk of death every 10 years than the increased risk per year, and that will be very much close to 1.
- Specify which type of *P*-value is quoted (e.g. LR or Wald test).
- Confirm that the assumptions for the logistic regression were met, in particular that the events are independent and the relationship plausibly loglinear. If the design is a matched one ensure that the analysis uses an appropriate method such as conditional logistic regression.
- Report any sensitivity analysis carried out.
- Name the statistical package used in the analysis. This is important because different packages sometimes have different definitions of common terms.
- Specify whether the explanatory variables were tested for interaction.

3.13 Reading about logistic regression

In addition to the points in Sections 1.11 and 2.10.
- Is logistic regression appropriate? Is the outcome a simple binary variable? If there is a time attached to the outcome then survival analysis might be better (Chapter 4).
- The outcome is often described as "relative risks". While this is often approximately true, they are better described as "approximate relative risks", or better "ORs". Note that for an OR, a non-significant result is associated with a 95% CI that includes 1 (not 0 as in multiple regression).
- Has a continuous variable been divided into two to create a binary variable for the analysis? How was the splitting point chosen? If it was chosen after the data had been collected, be very suspicious!
- Have any sensitivity tests been carried out? Is there evidence of overdispersion?
- If the design is a matched case–control study, has conditional logistic regression been carried out?

FREQUENTLY ASKED QUESTIONS

1 *Does it matter how the independent variable is coded?*
This depends on the computer package. Some packages will assume that any positive number is an event and 0 is a non-event. Changing the code from 0/1 to 1/0 will simply change the sign of the coefficient in the regression model.
2 *How is the OR associated with a continuous variable interpreted?*
The OR associated with a continuous variable is the ratio of odds of an event in two subjects, in which one subject is 1 unit higher than another. This assumes a linear model which can be hard to validate. One suggestion is to divide the data into five approximately equal groups, ordered on the continuous variable. Fit a model with four dummy variables corresponding to the four higher groups, with the lowest fifth as baseline. Look at the *coefficients* in the model (*not* the ORs). If they are plausibly increasing linearly, then a linear model may be reasonable. Otherwise, report the results of the model using the dummy variables.

EXERCISE

Reijman *et al.*[13] describe a cohort study of 1904 men and women with arthritis followed up for 6 years aged 55 years and over. They defined progression of hip osteoarthritis as a joint space narrowing of 1.0 mm or a total-hip replacement.
 They used logistic regression to analyse the data and got the following results

Predictor	OR (95% CI)
Age (years)	1.06 (1.04–1.08)
Sex (female)	1.8 (1.4–2.4)
Correctly predicted	89.7%

1 What are the possible problems with the outcome measure? What are the advantages?
2 If one person was 55 years old and another 65 years old at baseline, what are the increased odds of progression in the 65-year-old. What about a 75-year-old compared to a 65-year-old?
3 If 13% of men had progression, what percentage of women will have progressed?
4 If the dependent variable in this case is the log odds of hip progression, which of the models described in Figures 2.2–2.4 is this model analogous to?
5 Would you expect the model to correctly predict almost 90% of the group in another cohort? If not, why not?

References

1. Swinscow TDV, Campbell MJ. *Statistics at Square One*, 10th edn. London: BMJ Books, 2002.
2. Collett D. *Modelling Binary Data*, 2nd edn. London: Chapman and Hall/CRC Press, 2003.
3. Hosmer DW, Lemeshow S. *Applied Logistic Regression*, 2nd edn. New York: Wiley, 2000.
4. Julious SA, Mullee MA. Confounding and Simpson's Paradox. *Br Med J* 1994; **309:** 1480–1.
5. Lavie P, Herer P, Hoffstein V. Obstructive sleep apnoea syndrome as a risk factor for hypertension: population study. *Br Med J* 2000; **320:** 479–82.
6. Campbell MJ. Teaching logistic regression. In: Pereira-Mendoza L, Kea LS, Kee TW, Wong W-K, eds. *Statistical Education—Expanding the Network. Proceedings of the Fifth International Conference on Teaching Statistics.* Voorburg: ISI, 1998; 281–6.
7. Johnson CD, Toh SK, Campbell MJ. Combination of APACHE-II score and an obesity score (APACHE-O) for the prediction of severe acute pancreatitis. *Pancreatology* 2004; **4:** 1–6.
8. Altman DG, Machin D, Bryant TN, Gardner MJ, eds. *Statistics with Confidence.* London: BMJ Books, 2000.
9. Wald NJ, Nanchahal K, Thompson SG, Cuckle HS. Does breathing other people's tobacco smoke cause lung cancer? *Br Med J* 1986; **293:** 1217–22.
10. Breslow NE, Day NE. *Statistical Methods in Cancer Research 1: The Analysis of Case Control Studies.* Lyon: IARC, 1980.
11. Eason J, Markowe HLJ. Controlled investigation of deaths from asthma in hospitals in the North East Thames region. *Br Med J* 1987; **294:** 1255–8.
12. Churchill D, Allen J, Pringle M, Hippisley-Cox J, Ebdon D, Macpherson M, Bradley S. Consultation patterns and provision of contraception in general practice before teenage pregnancy: case control study. *Br Med J* 2000; **321:** 486–9.
13. Reijman M, Hazes JM, Pols HA, Bernsen RM, Koes B, *et al.* Role of radiography in predicting progression of osteoarthritis of the hip: prospective cohort study. *Br Med J* 2005; **330:** 1183–7.

Chapter 4 **Survival analysis**

Summary

When the dependent variable is a survival time, we need to allow for censored observations. We can display the data using a Kaplan–Meier plot. A useful model for modelling survival times on explanatory variables is known as a *proportional hazard* model, which is also referred to as a *Cox model*. It is a generalisation of the log-rank test, which is used for one binary independent variable, to allow for multiple independent variables that can be binary, categorical and continuous. It does not require a specification of an underlying survival distribution. A useful extension is to allow for stratification of an important categorical prognostic factor, so that subjects in different strata can have different underlying survival distributions.

4.1 Introduction

In survival analysis, the key variable is the time until some event. Commonly it is the time from treatment for a disease to death, but, in fact, it can be time to any event. Examples include time for a fracture to heal and time that a nitroglycerine patch stays in place. As for binary outcomes, we imagine individuals suffering an event, but attached to this *event* is a *survival time*.

There are two main distinguishing features about survival analysis:

1 The presence of *censored observations*. These can arise in two ways. Firstly, individuals can be removed from the data set, without suffering an event. For example, in a study looking at survival from some disease, they may be lost to follow-up, or get run over by a bus, and so, all we know is that they survived up to a particular point in time. Secondly, the study might be closed at a particular time point, as for example when a clinical trial is halted. Those still in the study are also regarded as censored, since they were alive when data collection was stopped. Clinical trials often recruit over a period of time, hence subjects recruited more recently will have less time to suffer an event than subjects recruited early on.

2 The development of models that do not require a particular distribution for the survival times, the so-called *semi-parametric models*. This methodology allows a great deal of flexibility, with fewer assumptions than are required for fully parametric models.

A critical assumption in these models is that the probability that an individual is censored is unrelated to the probability that the individual suffers an event. If individuals who respond poorly to a treatment are removed before death and treated as censored observations, then the models that follow are invalid. This is the so-called *uninformative* or *non-informative censoring* assumption.

The important benefit of survival analysis over logistic regression, say, is that the time an individual spent in the study can be used in the analysis, even if they did not suffer an event. In survival, the fact that one individual spent only 10 days in the study, whereas another spent 10 years is taken into account. In contrast, in a simple Chi-squared test or in logistic regression, all that is analysed is whether the individual suffered an event or not.

Further details are given in Collett,[1] and Parmar and Machin.[2]

4.2 The model

The dependent variable in survival analysis is what is known as the *hazard*. This is a probability of dying at a point in time, but it is conditional on surviving up to that point in time, which is why it is given a specific name.

Suppose we followed a cohort of 1000 people from birth to death. Say for the age group 45–54 years, there were 19 deaths. In a 10-year age group there are 10×1000 *person-years at risk*. We could think of the death rate per person-year for 45–54-year olds as $19/(10 \times 1000) = 1.9$ per 1000. However, if there were only 910 people alive by the time they reached 45 years of age, then the risk of death per person-year in the next 10 years, having survived to 45 years, is $19/(10 \times 910) = 2.1$ per 1000 per year. This is commonly called the *force of mortality*. In general, suppose X people were alive at the start of a year in a particular age group, and x people died during a period of width, t. The risk over that period is $x/(tX)$. If we imagine the width, t of the interval getting narrower, then the number of deaths x will also fall but the ratio x/t will stay constant. This gives us the *instantaneous death rate* or the *hazard rate* at a particular time. (An analogy might be measuring the speed of a car by measuring the time t it takes to cover a distance x from a particular point. By reducing x and t, we get the instantaneous speed at a particular point.)

The model links the hazard to an individual i at time t, $h_i(t)$ to a baseline hazard $h_0(t)$ by

$$\log_e[h_i(t)] = \log_e[h_0(t)] + \beta_1 X_{i1} + \cdots + \beta_p X_{ip} \tag{4.1}$$

where $X_{i1}, \ldots, X_{ip}$ are covariates associated with individual i.

This can also be written as

$$h_i(t) = h_0(t)\exp(\beta_1 X_{i1} + \cdots + \beta_p X_{ip}). \tag{4.2}$$

The baseline hazard $h_0(t)$ serves as a reference point, and can be thought of as an intercept β_0 in multiple regression equation (2.1). The important difference here is that it changes with time, whereas the intercept in multiple regression is constant. Similar to the intercept term, the hazard $h_0(t)$ in equation (4.1) represents the death rate for an individual whose covariates are all 0, which may be misleading if, say, age is a covariate. However, it is not important that these values are realistic, but that they act as a reference for the individuals in the study.

Model (4.1) can be contrasted with model (3.1), which used the logit transform, rather than the log. Unlike model (3.1), which yielded odds ratios (ORs), this model yields *relative risks*. Thus, if we had one binary covariate X, then $\exp(\beta)$ is the relative risk of (say) death for $X = 1$ compared to $X = 0$. Model (4.1) is used in *prospective* studies, where a relative risk can be measured.

This model was introduced by Cox[3] and is frequently referred to as the Cox regression model. It is called the proportional hazards model, because if we imagine two individuals, i and j, then (4.1) assumes that $h_i(t)/h_j(t)$ is constant over time; that is, even though $h_0(t)$ may vary, the two hazards for individuals whose covariates do not change with time remain proportional to each other. Since we do not have to specify $h_0(t)$, which is the equivalent of specifying a distribution for an error term, we have specified a model in (4.1) which contains parameters, and the model is sometimes described oxymoronically as *semi-parametric*.

Given a prospective study such as a clinical trial, imagine we chose at random an individual *who has suffered an event* and their survival time is T. For any time t the survival curve $S(t)$ is $P(T \geq t)$, that is the probability of a random individual surviving longer than t. If we assume there are no censored observations, then the estimate of $S(t)$ is just the proportion of subjects who survive longer than t. When some of the observations can be censored it is estimated by the *Kaplan–Meier* survival curve described in Swinscow and Campbell.[4] For any particular time t the hazard is

$$h(t) = \frac{P(T = t)}{P(T \geq t)}.$$

Suppose $S_0(t)$ is the baseline survival curve corresponding to a hazard $h_0(t)$, and $S_x(t)$ is the survival curve corresponding to an individual with covariates $X_{i1}, \ldots, X_{ip}$. Then it can be shown that under model (4.1),

$$S_x(t) = S_0(t)\exp(\beta_1 X_{i1} + \cdots + \beta_p X_{ip}). \tag{4.3}$$

This relationship is useful for checking the proportional hazards assumption, which we will show later.

The two important summary statistics are the number of events and the *person-years at risk*. There can only be one event per individual.

4.3 Uses of Cox regression

1 As a substitute for logistic regression when the dependent variable is a binary event, but where there is also information on the length of time to the event. This may be censored if the event does not occur.
2 To develop prognostic indicators for survival after operations, survival from disease or time to other events, such as time to heal a fracture.

4.4 Interpreting a computer output

The method of fitting model (4.1) is again a form of maximum likelihood, known as the *partial likelihood*. In this case, the method is quite similar to the matched case–control approach described in Chapter 3. Thus, one can consider any time at which an event has occurred, one individual (the case) has died and the remaining survivors are the controls. From model (4.1) one can write the probability that this particular individual is a case, given his/her covariates, compared to all the other survivors, and we attempt to find the coefficients that maximise this probability, for all the cases. Once again computer output consists of the likelihood, the regression coefficients and their standard errors (SEs). Swinscow and Campbell[4] describe the data given by McIllmurray and Turkie[5] on the survival of 49 patients with Dukes' C colorectal cancer. The data are given in Table 4.1.

It is important to appreciate that these are times from randomisation, or entry to the study. The first person in the table may have only entered the study 1 month before the investigator decided to stop the trial. The subjects with large censored survivals might have entered the study early, and have not suffered an event yet. In the computer, we have an "event" variable which takes the value 0 for a censored observation and 1 for an "event".

Table 4.1 Survival in 49 patients with Dukes' C colorectal cancer randomly assigned to either linolenic acid or control treatment (times with "+" are censored)

Treatment	Survival time (months)
γ-linolenic acid (*n* = 25)	1+, 5+, 6, 6, 9+, 10, 10, 10+, 12, 12, 12, 12, 12+, 13+, 15+,16+, 20+, 24, 24+, 27+, 32, 34+, 36+, 36+, 44+
Control (*n* = 24)	3+, 6, 6, 6, 6, 8, 8, 12, 12, 12+, 15+, 16+, 18+, 18+, 20, 22+, 24, 28+, 28+, 28+, 30, 30+, 33+, 42

The data are entered in the computer as:

Time	Event	Group (1 = γ-linolenic acid, 0 = control)
1	0	1
5	0	1
6	1	1
etc.		

The Kaplan–Meier survival curve is shown in Figure 4.1. Note the numbers at risk are shown on the graph. The output for the Cox regression is shown in Table 4.2.

Ties in the data occur when two survival times are equal. There are a number of ways of dealing with these. The most common is known as *Breslow's method*, and this is an approximate method that will work well when there are not too many ties. Some packages will also allow an "exact" method, but this usually takes more computer time. An "exact" partial likelihood is shown here, because the large number of ties in the data may render approximate methods less accurately.

From the output one can see that the hazard ratio associated with active treatment is 0.759 (95% CI 0.315 to 1.830). This has associated *P*-values of 0.54 by both the likelihood ratio (LR) and Wald methods, which implies that there is little evidence of efficacy. The risk and confidence interval (CI) are very similar to those given in Swinscow and Campbell[4] (Chapter 12 in *Statistics at Square One*, 10th edn), which used the log-rank test. An important point to note is that the z-statistic is *not* the ratio of the hazard ratio to its SE, but rather the ratio of the *regression coefficient* (log(hazard ratio)) to *its* SE (which is not given in this output).

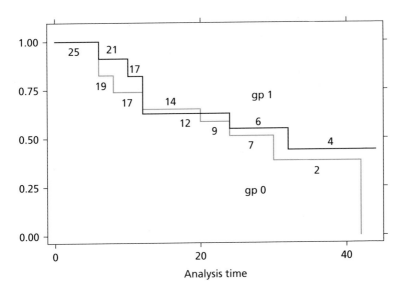

Figure 4.1 Kaplan–Meier survival plots for data in Table 4.1, where gp1 are those randomised to γ-linolenic acid, gp0 are those randomised to control, and the numbers are those at risk in each group.

Table 4.2 Analysis of γ-linolenic acid data

```
Cox regression — exact partial likelihood

No. of subjects   =          49     Number of obs  =        49
No. of failures   =          22
Time at risk      =         869
                                     LR chi2(1)     =      0.38
Log likelihood    =    -55.704161    Prob > chi2    =    0.5385
-----------------------------------------------------------------
 _t | Haz. Ratio Std.Err.    z     P>|z|   [95% Conf. Interval]
 _d |
----+------------------------------------------------------------
 gp | .7592211   .3407465  -0.614  0.539   .3150214      1.82977
-----------------------------------------------------------------
```

4.5 Survival analysis in action

Oddy et al.[6] looked at the association between breastfeeding and developing asthma in a cohort of children up to 6 years of age. The outcome was the age at developing asthma and they used Cox regression to examine the relationship with breastfeeding and to adjust for confounding factors: sex, gestational age, being of aboriginal descent and smoking in the household. They stated that "regression models were subjected to standard tests for goodness-of-fit including an investigation of the need for additional polynomial or interaction terms, an analysis of residuals, and tests of regression leverage and influence". They found that "other milk introduced before 4 months" was a risk factor for earlier asthma (hazard ratio 1.22, 95% CI 1.03 to 1.43, $P = 0.02$).

4.6 Interpretation of the model

In the model (4.1), the predictor variables can be continuous or discrete. If there is just one binary predictor variable X, then the interpretation is closely related to the log-rank test.[4] In this case, if the coefficient associated with X is b, then $\exp(b)$ is the *relative hazard* (often called the relative risk) for individuals for whom $X = 1$ compared with $X = 0$. When there is more than one covariate, then the interpretations are very similar to those described in Chapter 3 for binary outcomes. In particular, since the linear predictor is related to the outcome by an exponential transform, what is additive in the linear predictor becomes multiplicative in the outcome, as in logistic regression Section 3.4. In the asthma example, the risk of asthma of 1.22 for children exposed to other milk products before 4 months assumes all other covariates are held constant. The model assumes multiplicative risks so that if the risk of developing asthma early is double in boys, then boys exposed to other milk products before 4 months will be at $2 \times 1.22 = 2.44$ times the risk of girls not exposed to milk products.

4.7 Generalisations of the model

Suppose Oddy *et al.*[6] did not wish to assume that the incidence rate for aboriginal children was a constant multiple of the incidence rate of asthma for the non-aboriginal children. Then we can fit two separate models to the two groups:
(i) for the aboriginal children

$$\log_e[h_{iA}(t)] = \log_e[h_{0A}(t)] + \beta_1 X_{i1} + \cdots + \beta_p X_{ip}$$

(ii) and for the non-aboriginal children

$$\log_e[h_{iNA}(t)] = \log_e[h_{0NA}(t)] + \beta_1 X_{i1} + \cdots + \beta_p X_{ip}.$$

This is known as a *stratified Cox model*. Note that the regression coefficients, the βs – for the other covariates, sex, gestational age and smoking in household – are assumed to remain constant. This is an extension of the idea of fitting different intercepts for a categorical variable in multiple regression.

The model (4.1) assumes that the covariates are measured once at the beginning of the study. However, the model can be generalised to allow covariates to be time dependent. An example might be survival of a cohort of subjects exposed to asbestos, where a subject changes jobs over time and therefore changes his/her exposure to the dust. These are relatively easily incorporated into the computer analysis.

Another generalisation is to specify a distribution for $h_0(t)$ and use a fully parametric model. A common distribution is the *Weibull distribution*, which is a generalisation of the exponential distribution. This leads to what is known as an *accelerated failure time model*, and this is so called because the effect of a covariate X is to change the time scale by a factor $\exp(-\beta)$. Thus rather than, say, a subject dies earlier, one may think of them as simply living faster! Details of this technique are beyond the scope of this book, but it is becoming widely available on computer packages. Usually it will give similar answers to the Cox regression model.

4.8 Model checking

The assumption about linearity of the model is similar to that in multiple regression modelling described in Section 2.6 and can be checked in the same way. The methods for determining leverage and influence are also similar to those in multiple regression and hence we refer the reader to Section 2.7. There are a number of ways of calculating residuals, and various packages may produce some or all of *martingale residuals, Schoenfeld residuals* or *deviance residuals*. Details are beyond the scope of this book. However, since the Cox model is semi-parametric, the exact distribution of the residuals is unimportant. They can be used for checking outliers.

The new important assumption is that the hazard ratio remains constant over time. This is most straightforward when we have two groups to compare with no covariates. The simplest check is to plot the Kaplan–Meier survival curves for each group together. If they cross, then the proportional hazards assumption may be violated. For small data sets, where there may a great deal of error attached to the survival curve, it is possible for curves to cross, even under the proportional hazards assumption. However, it should be clear that an overall test of whether one group has better survival than the other is meaningless, when the answer will depend on the time that the test is made. A more sophisticated check is based on what is known as the *complementary log–log plot*. Suppose we have two groups with survival curves $S_1(t)$ and $S_2(t)$. We assume that the two groups are similar in all prognostic variables, except

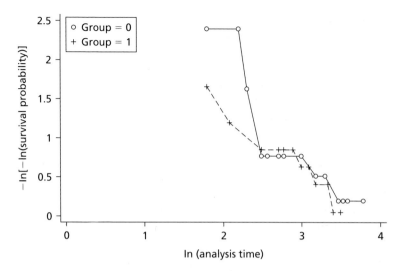

Figure 4.2 Log–log plot of survival curves in Figure 4.1.

group membership. From equations (4.1) and (4.3), if the proportional hazard assumption holds true, then

$$\log_e\{-\log_e[S_1(t)]\} = k + \log_e\{-\log_e[S_2(t)]\}$$

where k is a constant. This implies that if we plot both $\log_e\{-\log_e[S_1(t)]\}$ and $\log_e\{-\log_e[S_2(t)]\}$ against t, then the two curves will be parallel, with distance k apart.

This graph is plotted for the data in Table 4.1, and shown in Figure 4.2. The graph is, in fact, against $\log(t)$, but the principle of parallelism for proportional odds still holds. It can be seen that the two curves overlap considerably, but there is no apparent divergence between them, and so they are plausibly parallel.

There are also a number of formal tests of proportional hazards and further details are given in Parmar and Machin (pp. 176–7).[2] Most packages will provide a number of such tests. As an example, Table 4.3 shows the result of a test of proportional hazards, based on the Schoenfeld residuals and given by STATA.[7] It can be seen that this agrees with the intuitive graphical test that there is little evidence of a lack of proportional hazards.

The problems of testing proportional hazards are much more difficult when there are large number of covariates. In particular it is assumed that the proportional hazards assumption remains true for one variable independent of all the other covariates. In practice, most of the covariates will simply be potential confounders, and it is questionable whether statistical inference is

Table 4.3 Test of proportional hazards assumption (computer output)

```
Time: Time
- - - - - - - - - - - - - - - - - - - - - - - - - - - - - - - - - - - - - - - - -
             |        chi2 .        df           Prob>chi2
- - - - - - - -+- - - - - - - - - - - - - - - - - - - - - - - - - - - - - - - - -
global test  |        0.26          1              0.6096
- - - - - - - - - - - - - - - - - - - - - - - - - - - - - - - - - - - - - - - - -
```

advanced by assiduously testing each for proportionality in the model. It is important, however, that the main predictors, for example treatment group in a clinical trial, be tested for proportional hazards because it is impossible to interpret a fixed estimated relative risk if the true risk varies with time.

The other assumptions about the model are not testable from the data, but should be verified from the protocol. These include the fact that censoring is independent of an event happening. Thus in a survival study, one should ensure that patients are not removed from the study just before they die. Survival studies often recruit patients over a long period of time and so it is also important to verify that other factors remain constant over the period, such as the way patients are recruited into a study, and the diagnosis of the disease.

4.9 Reporting the results of a survival analysis

- Specify the nature of the censoring, and as far as possible validate that the censoring is non-informative.
- Report the total number of events, subjects and person-time of follow-up, with some measure of variability, such as a range for the latter. For a trial this should be done by a treatment group.
- Report an estimated survival rate at a given time, by group, with CIs.
- Display the Kaplan–Meier survival curves by group. To avoid misinterpretation of the right-hand end, terminate the curve when the number at risk is small, say 5. It is often useful to show the numbers at risk at regular time intervals, as shown in Figure 4.1. For large studies, this can be done at fixed time points, and shown just below the time axis.
- Specify the regression model used and note sensitivity analyses undertaken, and tests for proportionality of hazards.
- Specify a measure of risk for each explanatory variable, with a CI and a precise *P*-value. Note that these can be called relative risks, but it is perhaps better to refer to relative hazards.
- Report the computer program used for the analysis. Many research articles just quote Cox[3] without much evidence of having read that paper!

4.10   Reading about the results of a survival analysis

- Is the proportional hazards assumption reasonable and has it been validated?
- Are the conclusions critically dependent on the assumptions?
- In trials, are numbers of censored observations given by treatment group?

FREQUENTLY ASKED QUESTION

Does it matter how the event variable is coded?
Unlike logistic regression, coding an event variable 1/0 instead of 0/1 has a major effect on the analysis. Thus, it is vitally important to distinguish between the events (say deaths) and the censored times (say survivors). This is because, unlike ORs, hazard ratios are not symmetric to the coding and it matters if we are interested in survival or death. For example, if in two groups the mortality was 10% and 15%, respectively, we would say that the second group has a 50% increased mortality. However, the survival rates in the two groups are 90% and 85%, respectively, and so the second group has a 5/90 = 6% reduced survival rate.

EXERCISE 1

The table below is an analysis of some data given by Piantadosi.[8] It concerns survival of 76 patients with mesothelioma, and potential prognostic variables are age (years), sex (male/female), wtchg (weight change as a percentage), performance status (ps) (high or low) and five histologic subtypes. The analysis has been stratified by performance status, because it was felt that this may not have proportional hazards. Two models were fitted. One with age, sex and weight change, and the second including histological status as a set of dummy variables. The purpose of this analysis was to find significant prognostic factors for survival.

Model 1
```
Iteration 0:     log likelihood =-188.55165
Stratified Cox   regr. -- Breslow method for ties

No. of subjects  =          76          Number of obs  =      76
No. of failures  =          63
Time at risk     =       32380
                                         LR chi2 (A)    =    B
Log likelihood   =    -188.04719         Prob > chi2    = 0.7991
```

(continued)

```
  _t |
  _d |    Coef.    Std. Err.    z    P>|z|    [95% Conf. Interval]
-----+--------------------------------------------------------------
  age |   .0038245   .0128157   0.298   0.765   -.0212939    .0289429
wtchg |   .2859577   .3267412   0.875   0.381   -.3544433    .9263586
  sex |  -.1512113   .3102158     C     0.626      D           E
-------------------------------------------------------------------
                                              Stratified by ps
```

```
  _t |
  _d |  Haz. Ratio  Std. Err.    z    P>|z|    [95% Conf. Interval]
-----+--------------------------------------------------------------
  age |   1.003832   .0128648   0.298   0.765    .9789312    1.029366
wtchg |   1.331036   .4349043   0.875   0.381    .7015639    2.525297
  sex |    .859666   .266682      C     0.626       F           G
-------------------------------------------------------------------
                                              Stratified by ps
```

1 Fill in the missing values in the above output (A–G).

Model 2
```
Iteration 0:      log likelihood = -188.55165
Stratified Cox regr. -- Breslow method for ties

No. of subjects    =        76       Number of obs  =        76
No. of failures    =        63
Time at risk       =     32380
                                     LR chi2(7)     =     11.72
Log likelihood     =  -182.68981     Prob > chi2    =    0.1100
```

```
   _t |
   _d |  Haz. Ratio  Std. Err.    z    P>|z|   [95% Conf. Interval]
--------+--------------------------------------------------------------
    age |   .997813    .0130114  -0.168  0.867   .9726342    1.023644
  wtchg |   .9322795   .329234   -0.199  0.843   .4666001    1.86272
    sex |   .782026    .2646556  -0.727  0.468   .4028608    1.518055
Ihist_2 |   .7627185   .4007818  -0.515  0.606   .2723251    2.136195
Ihist_3 |   4.168391   2.87634    2.069  0.039   1.077975    16.11863
Ihist_4 |   .9230807   .5042144  -0.147  0.884   .3164374    2.692722
Ihist_5 |   5.550076   5.264405   1.807  0.071   .8647887    35.6195
----------------------------------------------------------------------
                                              Stratified by ps
```

1 What is the LR Chi-square for the histological type, with its degrees of freedom? Comment on its statistical significance.

2 What is the hazard ratio of dying for patients with histology type 2, compared to histology type 1, given they are of same gender, age and have same weight change, with a CI?

3 In model 2, what is the change in risk of dying for an individual relative to someone 10 years younger, given that they are of the same gender and histological type, and had same weight change?

EXERCISE 2

Campbell et al.[9] describe a cohort study over 24 years of 726 men exposed to slate dust and 529 controls. They used a Cox regression to examine the effect of slate dust exposure on mortality. They stratified by age group (10 years) in the analysis. They measured smoking habit and forced expiratory volume (FEV_1 a measure of lung function in litres) at baseline.

They found the following results:

		Hazard ratio	95% CI	P-value
Model 1	Slate	1.21	1.02 to 1.44	0.032
Model 2	Slate	1.24	1.04 to 1.47	0.015
	Smokers[a]	2.04	1.54 to 2.70	<0.001
	Ex-smokers[a]	1.46	1.07 to 1.98	0.016
Model 3	Slate	1.17	0.97 to 1.41	0.11
	Smokers[a]	1.96	1.44 to 2.67	<0.001
	Ex-smokers[a]	1.46	1.05 to 2.03	0.046
	FEV_1	0.74	0.65 to 0.83	<0.001

[a]Relative to non-smokers.

1 Describe the findings. Include in your explanation the reason for using a stratified analysis. Why do you think the hazard ratio for slate changes little when smoking habit is included in the model, and yet becomes non-significant when FEV_1 is included. State two major assumptions underlying *model 2* and how they might be tested. Interpret the coefficient for FEV_1 in *model 3*.

References

1. Collett D. *Modelling Survival Data in Medical Research*. London: Chapman and Hall, 1994.

2. Parmar MK, Machin D. *Survival Analysis: A Practical Approach*. Chichester: John Wiley, 1995.

3. Cox DR. Regression models and life tables (with discussion). *J Roy Statist Soc B* 1972; **34:** 187–220.
4. Swinscow TDV, Campbell MJ. *Statistics at Square One*, 10th edn. London: BMJ Books, 2002.
5. McIllmurray MB, Turkie E. Controlled trial of γ-linolenic acid in Duke's C colorectal cancer. *Br Med J* 1987; **294:** 1260; **295:** 475.
6. Oddy WH, Holt PG, Sly PD, Read AW, Landau LI, Stanley FJ, Kendall GE, Burton PR. Association between breast feeding and asthma in 6 year old children: findings of a prospective birth cohort study. *Br Med J* 1999; **319:** 815–19.
7. STATACorp. STATA Statistical Software Release 8.0. College Station, TX: Stata Corporation, 2003.
8. Piantadosi A. *Clinical Trials: A Methodologic Perspective*. Chichester: John Wiley, 1997.
9. Campbell MJ, Hodges NG, Thomas HF, Paul A, Williams JG. A 24 year cohort study of mortality in slate workers in North Wales. *J Occup Med* 2005; **55:** 448–53.

Chapter 5 **Random effects models**

Summary

Random effects models are useful in the analysis of *repeated measures* studies and *cluster randomised trials*, where the observations can be grouped, and within the group they are not independent. They are also useful in the analysis of *multi-centre trials* and in *meta-analysis*. Ignoring the correlation of observations within groups can lead to underestimation of the standard error (SE) of key estimates. There are two types of models: *cluster specific* and *marginal models*. Marginal models are easier to fit and utilise a technique known as *generalised estimating equations* (*gee*).

5.1 Introduction

The models described so far only have one error term. In multiple regression, as described by model (2.1) the error term was an explicit variable, ε, added to the predictor. In logistic regression, the error was Binomial and described how the observed and predicted values were related. However, possibilities are there for more than one error term. A simple example of this is when observations are repeated over time on individuals. There is then the random variation *within individuals* (repeating an observation on an individual does not necessarily give the same answer) and random variation *between individuals* (one individual differs from another). Another example would be the one in which each doctor treat a number of patients. There is *within-doctor variation* (since patients vary) and *between-doctor variation* (since different doctors are likely to have different effects). These are often known as *hierarchical data structures* since there is a natural hierarchy, with one set of observations nested within another. One form of model used to fit data of this kind is known as a *random effects model*. In recent years, there has been a great deal of interest in this type of model, and results are now regularly appearing in the medical literature. This chapter can no more than alert the reader to the importance of the topic.

5.2 Models for random effects

Consider a randomised trial, where there are single measurements on individuals, but the individuals form distinct groups, such as being treated by a particular doctor.

For continuous outcomes, y_{ij}, for an individual j in group i, we assume that

$$y_{ij} = \beta_0 + z_i + \beta_1 X_{1ij} + \cdots + \beta_p X_{pij} + \varepsilon_{ij}. \tag{5.1}$$

This model is very similar to equation (2.1), with the addition of an extra term z_i.

Here z_i is assumed to be a random variable with $E(z_i) = 0$, $\mathrm{Var}(z_i) = \sigma_B^2$ and reflects the overall effect of being in group i, and the X_{kij}s are the covariates on the kth covariate on the jth individual in the ith group with regression coefficients β_k.

We assume $\mathrm{Var}(\varepsilon_{ij}) = \sigma^2$, that z_i and ε_{ij} are uncorrelated and thus $\mathrm{Var}(y_{ij}) = \sigma^2 + \sigma_B^2$.

Thus, the variability of an observation has two components: the within- and the between-group variances.

The observations within a group are correlated and

$$\mathrm{Corr}(y_{ij}, y_{ik}) = \rho = \frac{\sigma_B^2}{\sigma^2 + \sigma_B^2} \quad \text{if } j \text{ and } k \text{ differ.}$$

This is known as the *intra-cluster (group) correlation* (ICC).

It can be shown that when a model is fitted, which ignores the z_is, the SE of the estimate of β_i is usually too small, and thus in general is likely to increase the Type I error rate. In particular, if all the groups are of the same size, m, then the variance of the estimate increases by $(1 + (m - 1)\rho)$ and this is known as the *design effect* (DE).

For some methods of fitting the model, we also need to assume that z_i and ε_{ij} are Normally distributed, but this is not always the case.

Model (5.1) is often known as the *random intercepts model*, since the intercepts are $\beta_0 + z_i$ for different groups i and these vary randomly. They are a subgroup of what is known as *multi-level models*, since the different error terms can be thought of as being different levels of a hierarchy, individuals nested within groups. They are also called *mixed models* because they mix random effects and fixed effects. Model (5.1) is called an *exchangeable model* because it would not affect the estimation procedure if two observations within a cluster were exchanged. Another way of looking at exchangeability, is that from equation (5.1), given a value for z_i, the correlation between y_{ij} and $y_{ij'}$ is the same for any individuals j and j' in the same group. Random effects models can be extended to the Binomial and Poisson models. As the random effect induces variability above that predicted by the model they are often called *over-dispersed* models. A common extension of the Poisson is the *negative Binomial*. Survival models can also be extended to include random effects, in which case the random effect is commonly known as the *frailty*.

Further details of these models are given in Brown and Prescott.[1] Repeated measures are described in Crowder and Hand,[2] and Diggle *et al.*[3] and the hierarchical models are described by Goldstein.[4]

5.3 Random vs fixed effects

Suppose we wish to include a variable in a model that covers differing groups of individuals. It could be a generic description, such as "smokers" or "non-smokers", or it could be quite specific, such as patients treated by Doctor A or Doctor B. The conventional method of allowing for categorical variables is to fit dummy variables as described in Chapter 2. This is known as a *fixed effect model*, as the effect of being in a particular group is assumed fixed, and represented by a fixed population parameter. Thus, "smoking" will decrease lung function by a certain amount on average. Being cared for by Doctor A may also affect your lung function, particularly if you are asthmatic. However, Doctor A's effect is of no interest to the world at large, in fact it is only so much extra noise in the study. However, the effect of smoking is of interest generally. The main difference between a fixed and a random effects model depends on the intention of the analysis. If the study were repeated, would the same groups be used again? If not, then a random effects model is appropriate. By fitting dummy variables we are removing the effect of the differing groups as confounders. However, if these groups are unique to this study, and in a new study there will be a different set of groups, then we are pretending accuracy that we do not have since the effects we have removed in the first study will be different in a second study. Thus, random effects are sources of "error" in a model due to individuals or groups over and above the unit "error" term and, in general, the SEs of the fixed components will be greater when a random component is added.

5.4 Use of random effects models

5.4.1 Cluster randomised trials

A cluster randomised trial is one in which groups of patients are randomised to an intervention or control rather than individual patients. The group may be a geographical area, a general or family practice, or a school. A general practice trial actively involves general practitioners and their primary health care teams, and the unit of randomisation may be the practice or health care professional rather than the patient. The effectiveness of the intervention is assessed in terms of the outcome for the patient.

There are many different features associated with cluster randomised trials and some of the statistical aspects were first discussed by Cornfield.[5] A useful discussion has been given by Zucker et al.[6] The main feature is that patients treated by one health care professional tend to be more similar than those treated by different health care professionals. If we know which doctor a patient is being treated by we can predict slightly better than by chance the performance of the patient and thus the observations for one doctor are not completely independent. What is surprising is how even a small correlation can greatly affect the design and analysis of such studies. For example with an ICC of 0.05 (a value commonly found in general practice trials), and 20 patients per group, the usual SE estimate for a treatment effect, ignoring the effect of clustering, will be about 30% lower than a valid estimate should be. This greatly increases the chance of getting a significant result even when there is no real effect (a Type I error).

Further discussion on the uses and problems of cluster randomised trials in general (family) practice has been given by Campbell.[7]

5.4.2 Repeated measures

A repeated measures study is where the same variable is observed on more than one occasion on each individual. An example might be a clinical trial to reduce blood pressure, where the blood pressure is measured 3, 6, 12 and 24 weeks after treatment. Each individual will have an effect on blood pressure, measured by the variable z_i. The individuals themselves are a sample from a population, and the level of blood pressure of a particular individual is not of interest.

A simple method of analysing data of this type is by means of summary measures.[8,9] Using this method we simply find a summary measure for each individual, often just the average, and analyse this as the primary outcome variable. This then eliminates the within-individual variability, and therefore we have only one error term, due to between-individual variation, to consider. Other summary values might be the maximum value attained over the time period, or the slope of the line. For repeated measures, the data are collected in order, and the order may be important. Model (5.1) can be extended to allow for the so-called *autoregressive models*, which take account of the ordering, but that is beyond the scope of this book.

5.4.3 Sample surveys

Another simple use of the models would be in a sample survey, for example to find out levels of depression in primary care. A random sample of practices is chosen and within them a random sample of patients. The effect of being cared for by a particular practice on an individual is not of prime interest. If we repeat the study we would have a different set of practices. However, the variation induced on the estimate of the proportion of depressed patients by different practices *is* of interest, as it will affect the confidence interval (CI). Thus, we need to allow for between-practice variation in our overall estimate.

5.4.4 Meta-analysis

Meta-analysis is used to combine results from different studies. It is commonly used to combine the results of different clinical trials of the same intervention and the same outcome. It can also be used to combine case–control studies. There are two sorts of meta-analysis: (i) which uses individual patient data and (ii) which uses summary measures, such as odds ratios (OR) from the different studies. The latter is more common, since access to individual data from a number of studies is rare.

In a meta-analysis, for each trial, i, we obtain an estimate of a treatment effect. For simplicity suppose it is a difference in means, d_i, but it could be an OR or a relative risk. Each trial will also report an SE for the estimate, ε_i. Then a simple random effects model is:

$$d_i = \beta_0 + z_i + \varepsilon_i. \qquad (5.2)$$

Here the β_0 is a measure of the average treatment effect and the z_i is a random term which allows the between trial variability in the estimate of the treatment difference to be accounted for in the overall estimate and its SE. However, this assumes that the individual trials are in some way representative of what would happen in a population, even though centres taking part in trials are not chosen at random. In addition, if there are few trials in the meta-analysis, the estimate of σ_B^2 will be poor. In meta-analysis, random effects "allow for" heterogeneity but do not "explain" it. Investigation of heterogeneity is an important aim in meta-analysis. It is wise to consult an experienced statistician for advice on these issues and there are some recent books on the subject.[10,11]

An example of a meta-analysis, not of trials but of case–control studies has already been described in Chapter 3 (Table 3.8). It is analysed there as a fixed effects model. However, the four case–control studies described there could be regarded as four samples from a larger pool of potential case–control studies, and hence a random effects model may seem appropriate. Here the z_i term would reflect the heterogeneity of the intervention effect over studies.

5.4.5 Multi-centre trials

Multi-centre trials enrol subjects from more than one site. They are useful for evaluating treatments of rare diseases, and also ensure reproducibility of the treatment effect across a broad range of characteristics that distinguish the sites. A useful analogy would be that of an individual patient data meta-analysis, where each centre can be regarded as a separate study. The crucial difference here is not just whether the treatment effect can be assumed random, but whether the centre effect itself is random (i.e. the centre affects the outcome for both the intervention and the control). Strictly speaking, centres should be considered a random effect only when they are selected randomly from a population of centres. In practice, of course, they are volunteers, with prior experience or a special interest in the disease or treatment. The use of random effects models here is somewhat controversial. If the number of centres is small (say <10), then modelling centres as either fixed or random can produce conflicting results, and the random effects models are more conservative. It is wise to consult an experienced statistician on these issues.[12]

5.5 Random effects models in action

5.5.1 Cluster trials
Diabetes from diagnosis was a study of patient-centred intervention for the treatment of newly diagnosed diabetics.[13] Briefly, 41 practices were recruited and randomised into two groups: 21 in the intervention and 20 in the comparison arm. In the intervention group the health professionals were given 1.5 days group training introducing the evidence for and skills of patient centred care. They were also given a patient-held booklet which encouraged asking questions. The other group were simply given the British Diabetic Association guidelines on the management of newly diagnosed diabetics. There were a number of outcomes such as the HbA1c, the body mass index (BMI) at 1 year after intervention and process measures such as patient satisfaction. The important points are that patients treated by a particular doctor will tend to have more similar outcomes than patients treated by different doctors, and the trial is of an intervention package that would be given to different doctors in any future implementation. The effect of the intervention was a difference in BMI at 1 year of $1.90 \, kg/m^2$ in the two groups (SE 0.82). With no allowance for clustering the SE was 0.76, which magnifies the apparent significance of the effect.

5.5.2 Repeated measures
Doull *et al.*[14] looked at the growth rate of 50 children with asthma before and after taking inhaled steroids. They showed that, compared to before treatment, the difference in growth rate between weeks 0 and 6 after treatment was $-0.067 \, mm/week$ (95% CI -0.12 to -0.015), whereas at weeks 19–24, compared to before treatment, it was -0.002 (95% CI -0.054 to 0.051). This showed that the growth suppressive action of inhaled corticosteroids is relatively short lived. The random effects model enabled a random child effect to be included in the model. It allowed differing numbers of measurements per child to be accounted for. The model gives increased confidence that the results can be generalised beyond these particular children.

5.5.3 Meta-analysis

Pickup et al.[15] looked at 11 trials comparing a continuous subcutaneous insulin infusion delivered by a pump against optimised insulin therapy in patients with Type 1 diabetes. They standardised the outcome (HbA1c) by dividing by the standard deviation in each trial, to allow for different methods of measuring HbA1c. Using a random effects model, they found the standardised mean difference between the two treatments to be 0.44 (95% CI 0.20 to 0.63). This is equivalent to 0.51% in the original units. They found a fixed effects model gave a similar standardised mean difference to the random effects model (0.41) but with slightly narrower CI (0.23 to 0.58).

A good way to summarise a meta-analysis is via a *forest plot* which is a plot of the estimates and CIs. An example is given in Figure 5.1, which is a meta-analysis of 28 trials of iron supplementation for the prevention of infections in children.[16] The outcome measure is the incidence rate ratio (IRR) (the relative risk, discussed in Chapter 6). This is a good illustration of the meaning of random effects. Each CI is a measure of within-study variation; the wider CIs are associated with the smaller studies. This is modelled by the term ε_i in equation (5.2). The variation of the point estimates is a measure of between-study variation, which is modelled by the z_i in equation (5.2). The test of heterogeneity given at the bottom of the figure is a test of whether the between- and within-study variation are commensurate. One can see from the P-value that they are not; there is more variation between studies than would be expected if they were all sampled from the same population. The "pooled" estimate, the last CI on the plot, is estimated using a random effects model. In this case one can see that the CI includes unity, suggesting no real effect of iron supplementation on the incidence of infections.

One problem with meta-analysis is a *publication bias*. This occurs when studies with small effects are not published. One way of investigating this is to plot a measure of precision on the y-axis (the inverse of the SE, or the sample size), and a measure of effect on the x-axis (a difference in means, a log OR or a log risk ratio). This is known as a *funnel* plot. If the studies are truly representative one would expect that the effect measures would be symmetrically distributed around a central point, so that small effects are as equally represented as large effects. The central point would have the highest precision so that the distribution would appear like an inverted funnel. A lack of symmetry would suggest publication bias. An example of a funnel plot is given in Figure 5.2 from the study by Gera and Sachdev.[16] One can see that the plot is reasonable symmetrical and the studies with the highest precision (smallest SE) are clustered around the central value which is close to 0. The authors concluded from this that there was little evidence of publication bias.

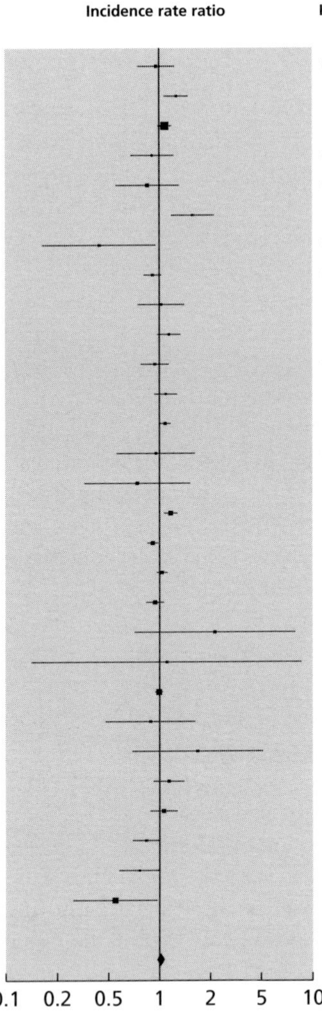

	Episodes of infection/child years		Incidence rate ratio	Incidence rate ratio exact 95% CI
	Iron	Control		
James	96/77	116/89		0.96 (0.72 to 1.26)
Brusner	256/57	254/73		1.29 (1.08 to 1.54)
Fuerth	1007/494	773/410		1.08 (0.98 to 1.19)
Menendez 1	75/118	81/114		0.89 (0.64 to 1.23)
Menendez 2	36/149	42/154		0.34 (0.52 to 1.34)
Hombergh	107/13	65/13		1.65 (1.20 to 2.28)
Angeles	9/7	21/6		0.41 (0.16 to 0.93)
Power	469/53	460/47		0.90 (0.79 to 1.03)
Palupi	71/16	69/16		1.04 (0.74 to 1.47)
Rosado 1	285/54	255/56		1.16 (0.98 to 1.38)
Rosado 2	202/55	211/54		0.94 (0.77 to 1.15)
Javaid	432/58	189/28		1.10 (0.93 to 1.32)
Berger	1328/75	1178/73		1.09 (1.01 to 1.18)
Lawless	26/11	26/11		0.95 (0.53 to 1.71)
Irigoyen	20/114	13/53		0.72 (0.34 to 1.56)
Oppenheimer	1027/197	921/208		1.18 (1.08 to 1.29)
Singhal	889/122	2001/248		0.91 (0.84 to 0.98)
Mitra	1375/134	1420/144		1.04 (0.96 to 1.12)
Hemminki	504/164	521/158		0.94 (0.82 to 1.06)
Agarwal	12/4	5/4		2.29 (0.75 to 8.30)
Nagpal	3/5	3/5		1.11 (0.15 to 8.30)
Rice	2781/268	2798/267		0.99 (0.94 to 1.05)
Idjradinata	19/8	21/8		0.87 (0.44 to 1.69)
Smith	14/27	8/27		1.77 (0.69 to 4.86)
Adam	176/108	146/103		1.15 (0.92 to 1.44)
Gabresellasie	219/188	206/188		1.06 (0.87 to 1.29)
Atukorala 1	297/21	147/9		0.82 (0.67 to 1.01)
Atukorala 2	137/22	70/8		0.73 (0.54 to 0.99)
Cantwell	15/188	44/288		0.52 (0.27 to 0.96)
Pooled	4027/2802	3865/2848		1.02 (0.96 to 1.08)

0.1 0.2 0.5 1 2 5 10

Heterogeneity Q = 78.29, df = 28, $P < 0.0001$

Figure 5.1 A forest plot for the IRR for trials on iron supplementation in children for all infectious diseases from Gera and Sachdev[16] (reproduced with permission).

5.6 Ordinary least squares at the group level

Cornfield[5] stated that one should "analyse as you randomise". Since randomisation is at the level of the group, a simple analysis would be to calculate "summary measures", such as the mean value for each group, and analyse these as the primary outcome variable.

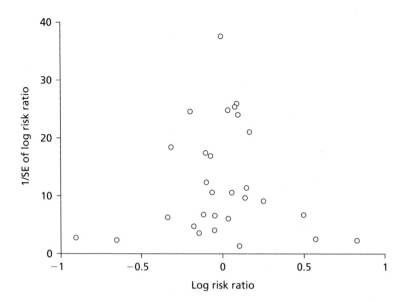

Figure 5.2 A funnel plot of the meta-analysis from Gera and Sachdev[16] (reproduced with permission).

Omitting the covariates from the model for simplicity, except for a dummy variable δ_i which takes the value 1 for the intervention and 0 for the control, it can be shown that:

$$\bar{y}_i = \mu + \tau\delta_i + \bar{\varepsilon}_i \tag{5.3}$$

where $\bar{y}_i$ is the mean value for the n_i individuals with outcome $y_{ij}, j = 1, \ldots, n_i$ for group i and

$$\operatorname{Var}(\bar{y}_i) = \sigma_B^2 + \frac{\sigma^2}{n_i}. \tag{5.4}$$

Equation (5.3) is a simple model with independent errors, which are homogeneous if each n_i is of similar size. An ordinary least squares estimate at group level of τ is unbiased and the SE of estimate is valid provided the error term is independent of the treatment effect.

Thus, a simple analysis at the group level would be the following: if each n_i is the same or not too different carry out a two-sample t-test on the group level means. This is the method of summary measures mentioned in Section 5.4.2. It is worth noting that if σ^2 is 0 (all values from a group are the same) then group size does not matter. An alternative method of analysis is to carry out a weighted analysis using as weights the inverse of the variance in equation (5.4). (Given data x_i ($i = 1...n$) and a set of weights w_i a weighted mean is given by $\bar{x}_{\text{weighted}} = \sum_i w_i x_i / \sum_i w_i$). The terms σ_B^2 and σ^2 can be estimated using an analysis of variance. If σ_B^2 can be assumed 0 the weights are simply the inverse of the sample sizes. This is the *fixed effect* analysis.

There are a number of problems with a group-level approach. The main one is how should individual level covariates be allowed for? It is unsatisfactory to use group averaged values of the individual-level covariates. This method ignores the fact that the summary measures may be estimated with different precision for different individuals. The advantage of random effects models over summary measures is that they can allow for covariates which may vary with individuals. They also allow for different numbers of individuals per group.

5.7 Computer analysis

5.7.1 Likelihood and gee
Many computer packages will now fit random effects models although different packages may use different methods of fitting model (5.1). The likelihood method first assumes a distribution (usually Normal) for each z_i and then formulates a probability of observing each y_{ij} conditional on each z_i. Using the distribution of each z_i we can obtain an expected probability over every possible z_i. This involves mathematical integration and is difficult. Since the method calculates the regression coefficients separately for each group or cluster, this is often known as the *cluster specific model*. A simpler method is known as *generalised estimating equations* (*gee*) which does not require Normality of the random effects. This method essentially uses the mean values per group as the outcome, and adjusts the SE for the comparison to allow for within group correlation using the *robust or sandwich estimator* described in Appendix 3. The gee methodology is based on what is known as a *marginal model*. In an ordinary table of data, the edges of the table are the margins and they contain the mean values; hence the name marginal model. The gee methodology uses the means per group, with the correlations within a group as a nuisance factor. As the group is the main item for analysis, gee methodology may be unreliable unless the number of clusters exceeds 20, and preferably 40.

The methods can be extended to allow for Binomial errors, so that one can get random effect logistic regression. The maximum likelihood method is less likely to be available in computer packages for logistic regression, and many packages at present only offer gee methods. This type of model is generalised quite naturally to a Bayesian approach (see Appendix 4). This is beyond the scope of this book but further details are given in Turner *et al.*[17]

5.7.2 Interpreting computer output

Table 5.1 gives some data which are a subset of data from Kinmonth et al.[13] They consist of the BMI at 1 year on a number of patients in 10 practices, under one of two treatment groups.

The results are shown in Table 5.2. Table 5.2(i) shows the results of fitting an ordinary regression without clustering, which yields an estimate of a

Table 5.1 Data on BMI[13]

Subject	BMI (kg/m^2)	Treat	Practice
1	26.2	1	1
2	27.1	1	1
3	25.0	1	2
4	28.3	1	2
5	30.5	1	3
6	28.8	1	4
7	31.0	1	4
8	32.1	1	4
9	28.2	1	5
10	30.9	1	5
11	37.0	0	6
12	38.1	0	6
13	22.1	0	7
14	23.0	0	7
15	23.2	0	8
16	25.7	0	8
17	27.8	0	9
18	28.0	0	9
19	28.0	0	10
20	31.0	0	10

Table 5.2 Computer output fitting regression models to data in Table 5.1

(i) Regression not allowing for clustering

```
  Source |       SS       df       MS              Number of obs  =     20
---------+------------------------------           F(1, 18)       =    0.05
   Model |  .881999519     1    .881999519         Prob > F       =  0.8279
Residual |  326.397937    18    18.1332187         R-squared      =  0.0027
---------+------------------------------           Adj R-squared  = -0.0527
   Total |  327.279937    19    17.2252598         Root MSE       =  4.2583

---------------------------------------------------------------------------
     bmi |    Coef.   Std. Err.      t    P > |t|    [95% Conf.   Interval]
---------+-----------------------------------------------------------------
   treat | .4199999   1.904375    0.221   0.828    -3.580943    4.420943
   _cons |    28.39   1.346596   21.083   0.000     25.56091    31.21909
---------------------------------------------------------------------------
```

(continued)

Table 5.2 (*continued*)

(ii) Regression with robust SEs

```
                                    Number of obs    =        20
                                    F( 1,  9)        =      0.02
                                    Prob > F         =    0.8789
                                    R-squared        =    0.0027
Number of clusters (group) = 10     Root MSE         =    4.2583
```

bmi	Coef.	Robust Std. Err.	t	P > |t|	[95% Conf.	Interval]
treat	.4199999	2.679838	0.16	0.879	-5.642215	6.482215
_cons	28.39	2.516677	11.28	0.000	22.69688	34.08312

(iii) Maximum likelihood random effects model

```
Fitting constant-only model:
Iteration 0:  log likelihood = -51.281055
Iteration 4:  log likelihood = -49.644194

Fitting full model:
Iteration 0:  log likelihood = -51.269825
Iteration 4:  log likelihood = -49.631613
```

```
Random-effects ML regression     Number of obs    =        20
Group variable (i) : group       Number of groups =        10

Random effects u_i ~ Gaussian    Obs per group: min =        1
                                              avg  =       2.0
                                              max  =         3

                                 LR chi2(1)       =      0.03
Log likelihood = -49.631613      Prob > chi2      =    0.8740
```

bmi	Coef.	Std. Err.	z	P > |z|	[95% Conf.	Interval]
treat	.3916501	2.467672	0.159	0.874	-4.444899	5.228199
_cons	28.39	1.740882	16.308	0.000	24.97793	31.80207
/sigma_u	3.737395	.9099706	4.107	0.000	1.953885	5.520904
/sigma_e	1.539626	.3430004	4.489	0.000	.8673579	2.211895
rho	.854917	.0848639			.6286473	.9630508

```
Likelihood ratio test of sigma_u=0: chi2(1) = 13.34
Prob > chi2 = 0.0003
```

(*continued*)

Table 5.2 (*continued*)

(iv) Generalised estimating equation

```
Iteration 1: tolerance = .01850836
Iteration 2: tolerance = .0000438
Iteration 3: tolerance = 1.029e-07
```

GEE population-averaged model				Number of obs	=	20
Group variable:		group		Number of groups	=	10
Link:		identity		Obs per group: min	=	1
Family:		Gaussian		avg	=	2.0
Correlation:		exchangeable		max	=	3
				Wald chi2(1)	=	0.02
Scale parameter:		18.1336		Prob > chi2	=	0.8803

bmi	Coef.	Std. Err.	z	P > |z|	[95% Conf.	Interval]
treat	.3937789	2.613977	0.151	0.880	-4.729523	5.51708
_cons	28.39	1.844712	15.390	0.000	24.77443	32.00557

(v) Regression on group means

Between regression (regression on group means)			Number of obs	=	20
Group variable (i) : group			Number of groups	=	10
R-sq: within = .			Obs per group: min	=	1
between = 0.0027			avg	=	2.0
overall = 0.0027			max	=	3
			F(1,8)	=	0.02
sd(u_i + avg(e_i.)) = 4.34548			Prob > F	=	0.8860

bmi	Coef.	Std. Err.	t	P > |t|	[95% Conf.	Interval]
treat	.4066669	2.748323	0.148	0.886	-5.930976	6.74431
_cons	28.39	1.943358	14.609	0.000	23.90861	32.87139

treatment effect of 0.42, with SE 1.90. As was stated earlier, since this ignores the clustering inherent in the data the SE will be too small. Table 5.2(ii) shows the results of fitting the model using robust standard errors, which are described in Appendix 3. One can see that the estimate of the treatment effect is the same but the SE is estimated as 2.68, which is much greater than in model (i). The robust standard error methods allows for heterogeneity in the variances between and within subjects. It also effectively weights the cluster means with the sample size of the cluster giving the same mean as the unweighted estimate. The maximum likelihood model weights the estimates depending on the within and between cluster variances and yields an estimate of the treatment effect of 0.39, with SE 2.47. This estimate will be different if (possibly by chance) the estimate of an effect is (say) larger for larger clusters. If there is no real association between size of effect and size of cluster, then for large samples the methods will give similar results. Usually it is reasonable to assume no association, but one might imagine that (say) a teaching method is more effective if a group is small. Note again how the SE is inflated compared to the model that fails to allow for clustering. The program also gives an estimate of the ICC coefficient, rho, of 0.85 and the between and within groups standard deviations, here denoted sigma_u (an estimate of our σ_B^2) and sigma_e (and estimate of our σ^2). The output also states the random effects are assumed Gaussian, which is a synonym for Normal (after C.F. Gauss, a German mathematician who first described the distribution). Using the method of gee, given in Table 5.2(iv), also yields a treatment estimate of 0.39, but an SE of 2.61. As described earlier, the assumption underlying the analyses in (ii), (iii) and (iv) is that individuals within a group are *exchangeable*. The estimate from gee can be contrasted with the method which uses the average per group (a summary measure) as the outcome in Table 5.2(v). This yields an estimate of 0.41, with an even larger SE of 2.74. This method does not weight the cluster means differently, so a small cluster will contribute the same as a large cluster.

The methods will give increasingly different results as the variation between groups increases. In this example the estimate of the treatment effect is quite similar for each method, but the SEs vary somewhat. Which method to choose will depend on factors such as the number of clusters and the size of each cluster. Any method which allows for clustering is acceptable. If the methods give markedly different results then this should be investigated. It can occur, for example, if there is a clear relation between effect size and cluster size.

5.8 Model checking

Most of the assumptions for random effects models are similar to those of linear or logistic models described in Chapters 2 and 3. The main difference is in the assumptions underlying the random term. Proper checking is beyond the scope of this book, but the maximum likelihood method assumes that the random terms are distributed Normally. If the numbers of measurements per cluster are fairly uniform, then a simple check would be to examine the cluster means, in a histogram. This is difficult to interpret if the numbers per cluster vary a great deal. In cluster randomised trials, it would be useful to check that the numbers of patients per cluster is not affected by treatment. Sometimes, when the intervention is a training package, for example, the effect of training is to increase recruitment to the trial, so leading to an imbalance in the treatment and control arms.

5.9 Reporting the results of random effects analysis

- Give the number of *groups* as well as the number of individuals.
- In a cluster randomised trial, give the group level means of covariates by treatment arm, so the reader can see if the trial is balanced *at a group level*.
- Describe whether a cluster specific or a marginal model is being used and justify the choice.
- Indicate how the assumptions underlying the distribution of the random effects were verified.
- Cluster randomised trials and meta-analyses now both have respective CONSORT statements to help report these areas.[18,19]

5.10 Reading about the results of random effects analysis

- What is the main unit of analysis? Does the statistical analysis reflect this? Repeating a measurement on one individual is not the same as making the second measurement on a different individual, and the statistical analysis should be different in each situation.
- In a meta-analysis, would a fixed effects or random effects model have been better?
- If the study is a cluster randomised trial, was an appropriate model used?
- If the analysis uses gee methodology, are there sufficient groups to justify the results?

FREQUENTLY ASKED QUESTIONS

1 *Given the plethora of methods that can be used to analyse random effects model, which should I use?*
This will depend on a number of factors, such as availability of software, and size of sample. One is warned not to use gee methods if the number of clusters is less than about 20. If the numbers of subjects per cluster is similar then all methods will produce similar results. A key question is whether the treatment effect varies with the cluster size. This could be investigated by trying several methods which weight the estimates differently and see if they give markedly different results. If they do differ, then the reasons should be investigated.

(continued)

2 *Should I use a fixed or random effects model in a meta-analysis?*
Following the advice of Whitehead[11] (p. 153) the choice should not be made
solely on whether the test for heterogeneity is significant. We need to
consider additional criteria such as the number of trials and the distribution of
the summary measures. With a small number of trials it is difficult to estimate
between trial variability, and if the results from the trials appear consistent,
then a fixed effects model may be more appropriate. If however, there are a
large number of trials, then a random effects model should be more
generalisable. It may be useful to fit both, and if the heterogeneity is low, the
results from the fixed and random models will agree. This was the approach
adopted b Pickup *et al.*, for example.[15] If the results differ then further
investigation is warranted.

EXERCISE

In Table 5.1 the mean values (kg/m^2) per practice were:
  Treatment 1: 26.65, 26.65, 30.5, 30.63, 29.55
  Treatment 2: 37.55, 22.55, 24.45, 27.9, 29.5
  Estimate the treatment effect (difference in treatment means) using
weights:

1 n_i
2 inverse of variance given by equation (5.4) (use estimates sigma_u and
   sigma_e given in Table 5.2(ii)).
3 equal weights.
4 Comment on possible outliers.

References

1. Brown H, Prescott R. *Applied Mixed Models in Medicine*. Chichester: John Wiley,
   1999.
2. Crowder M, Hand DJ. *Analysis of Repeated Measures*. London: Chapman and Hall,
   1999.
3. Diggle PJ, Heagerty P, Liang K-Y, Zeger S. *Analysis of Longitudinal Data*, 2nd
   edn. Oxford: Oxford Science Publications, 2002.
4. Goldstein H. *Multi-level Models*, 2nd edn. London: Arnold, 1996.
5. Cornfield J. Randomization by group: a formal analysis. *Am J Epidemiol* 1978;
   108: 100–2.

6. Zucker DM, Lakatos E, Webber LS, *et al.* Statistical design of the Child and Adolescent Trial for Cardiovascular Health (CATCH): implications of cluster randomization. *Controlled Clin Trials* 1995; **16:** 96–118.

7. Campbell MJ. Cluster randomised trials in general (family) practice. *Stat Methods Med Res* 2000; **9:** 81–94.

8. Matthews JNS, Altman DG, Campbell MJ, Royston JP. Analysis of serial measurements in medical research. *Br Med J* 1990; **300:** 230–5.

9. Campbell MJ, Machin D. *Medical Statistics: A Commonsense Approach*, 3rd edn. Chichester: John Wiley, 1999.

10. Sutton AJ, Abrams KR, Jones DR, Sheldon TA, Song F. *Methods for Meta-analysis in Medical Research.* Chichester: John Wiley, 2000.

11. Whitehead A. *Meta-analysis of Controlled Clinical Trials.* Chichester: John Wiley, 2002.

12. Senns S. Some controversies in planning and analyzing multi-center trials. *Stat Med* 1998; **17:** 1753–65.

13. Kinmonth AL, Woodcock A, Griffin S, Spiegal N, Campbell MJ. Randomised controlled trial of patient centred care of diabetes in general practice: impact on current wellbeing and future disease risk. *Br Med J* 1998; **317:** 1202–8.

14. Doull IJM, Campbell MJ, Holgate ST. Duration of growth suppressive effects of regular inhaled corticosteroids. *Arch Dis Child* 1998; **78:** 172–3.

15. Pickup J, Mattock M, Kerry S. Glycaemic control with continuous subcutaneous insulin infusion compared with intensive insulin injections in patients with type 1 diabetes: meta-analysis of randomised controlled trials. *Br Med J* 2002; **324:** 1–6.

16. Gera T, Sachdev HP. Effect of iron supplementation on incidence of infectious illness in children: a systematic review. *Br Med J* 2002; **325:** 1142–51.

17. Turner RM, Omar RZ, Thompson SG. Bayesian methods of analysis for cluster randomised trials with binary outcome data. *Stat Med* 2001; **20:** 453–72.

18. http://www.consort-statement.org/QUOROM

19. Campbell MK, Elbourne D, Altman DG. CONSORT statement: extension to cluster randomised trials. *Br Med J* 2004; **328:** 702–8.

Chapter 6 **Other models**

Summary

This chapter will consider three other regression models which are of considerable use in medical research: *Poisson regression, ordinal regression* and *time series regression*. Poisson regression is useful when the outcome variable is a count. Ordinal regression is useful when the outcome is ordinal, or ordered categorical. Time series regression is mainly used when the outcome is continuous, but measured together with the predictor variables serially over time.

6.1 Poisson regression

Poisson regression is an extension of logistic regression where the risk of an event to an individual is small, but there are a large number of individuals, so the number of events in a group is appreciable. We need to know not just whether an individual had an event, but for how long they were followed up, the *person-years*. This is sometimes known as the amount of time they were *at risk*. It is used extensively in epidemiology, particularly in the analysis of cohort studies. For further details see McNeil.[1]

6.1.1 The model
The outcome for a Poisson model is a count of events in a group, usually over a period of time, for example number of deaths over 20 years in a group exposed to asbestos. It is a *discrete quantitative variable* in the terminology of Chapter 1. The principal covariate is a measure of the amount of time the group have been in the study. Subjects may have been in the study for differing length of times (known as the *at risk period*) and so we record the time each individual is observed to give an exposure time e_i. In logistic regression we modelled the probability of an event π_i. Here we model the underlying rate λ_i which is the number of events expected to occur over a period i, E_i, divided by the time e_i. Instead of a logistic transform we use a simple log transform.

The model is

$$\log_e(\lambda_i) = \log_e\left(\frac{E_i}{e_i}\right) = \beta_0 + \beta_1 X_{i1} + \cdots + \beta_p X_{ip}. \qquad (6.1)$$

This may be rewritten as:

$$E_i = \exp[\log_e(e_i) + \beta_0 + \beta_1 X_{i1} + \cdots + \beta_p X_{ip}]. \qquad (6.2)$$

It is assumed that risk of an event rises directly with e_i and so in the model (6.2) the coefficient for $\log_e(e_i)$ is fixed at 1. This is known as an *offset* and is a special type of independent variable whose regression coefficient is fixed at unity.

Note that, as for the logistic regression, the *observed counts* have not yet appeared in the model. They are linked to the expected counts by the Poisson distribution (see Appendix 2). Thus we assume that the observed count y_i is distributed as a Poisson variable with parameter $E_i = \lambda_i e_i$.

Instead of a measure of the person-years at risk, we could use the predicted number of deaths, based on external data. For example, we could use the age/sex specific death rates for England and Wales to predict the number of deaths in each group. This would enable us to model the *standardised mortality ratio* (SMR). For further details see Breslow and Day.[2]

6.1.2 Consequences of the model

Consider a cohort study in which the independent variable is a simple binary 0 or 1, respectively, for people not exposed or exposed to a hazard. The dependent variable is the number of people who succumb to disease and also included in the model is the length of time they were on study. Then the coefficient b estimated from the model is the log of the ratio of the estimated incidence of the disease in those exposed and not exposed. Thus $\exp(b)$ is the estimated *incidence rate ratio* (IRR) or *relative risk*. Note that for prospective studies the relative risk is a more natural parameter than an odds ratio (OR). One can also use Poisson regression when the outcome is binary, in other words when the data can be summarised in a 2×2 table relating input to output. The structure of the model is such that $\exp(b)$ still estimates the relative risk, without invoking the Poisson assumption. However, as the Poisson assumption is not met, the standard errors (SEs) are incorrect. Recently Zou has demonstrated a method of obtaining valid estimates using *robust SEs*.[3]

6.1.3 Interpreting a computer output: Poisson regression for counts

The data layout is exactly the same as for the grouped logistic regression described in Chapter 3. The model is fitted by maximum likelihood.

Table 6.1 gives data from the classic cohort study of coronary deaths and smoking among British male doctors,[4] quoted in Breslow and Day,[2] and McNeil.[1]

Here the question is what is the risk of deaths associated with smoking, allowing for age? Thus the dependent variable is number of deaths per age per smoking group. Smoking group is the causal variable, age group is a confounder and the person-years is the offset. The analysis is given in Table 6.2.

Table 6.1 Coronary deaths from British male doctors

Deaths (D)	Person-years	Smoker	Age group at start study	Expected (E)	$\dfrac{(D-E)}{\sqrt{E}}$
32	52 407	1	35–44	27.2	0.92
2	18 790	0	35–44	6.8	−1.85
104	43 248	1	45–54	98.9	0.52
12	10 673	0	45–54	17.1	−1.24
206	28 612	1	55–64	205.3	0.05
28	5712	0	55–64	28.7	−0.14
186	12 663	1	65–74	187.2	−0.09
28	2585	0	65–74	26.8	0.23
102	5317	1	75–84	111.5	−0.89
31	1462	0	75–84	21.5	2.05

Table 6.2 Results of Poisson regression on data in Table 6.1

```
Iteration 0: log likelihood = -33.823578
Iteration 1: log likelihood = -33.60073
Iteration 2: log likelihood = -33.600412
Iteration 3: log likelihood = -33.600412

Poisson regression                    Number of obs   =        10
                                      LR chi2(5)      =    922.93
                                      Prob > chi2     =    0.0000
Log likelihood = -33.600412           Pseudo R2       =    0.9321

-----------------------------------------------------------------
       y |     IRR  Std. Err.    z   P>|z|  [95% Conf. Interval]
---------+-------------------------------------------------------
  smoker | 1.425664  .1530791 3.303  0.001  1.155102    1.7596
Age 45-54|  4.41056  .860515  7.606  0.000  3.008995  6.464962
Age 55-64| 13.83849 2.542506 14.301  0.000   9.65384  19.83707
Age 65-74| 28.51656 5.269837 18.130  0.000  19.85162  40.96364
Age 75-84| 40.45104 7.77548  19.249  0.000  27.75314  58.95862
    pyrs | (exposure)
-----------------------------------------------------------------
```

The five age groups have been fitted using four dummy variables, with age group 35–44 as the baseline. The model used here assumes that the relative risk of coronary death for smokers remains constant for each age group. The estimated relative risk for smokers compared to non-smokers is 1.43, with 95% confidence interval (CI) 1.16 to 1.76 which is highly significant ($P = 0.001$). Thus male British doctors are 40% more likely to die of a coronary death if they smoke. The LR Chi-square is an overall test of the model and is highly significant, but this significance is largely due to the age categories – coronary risk is highly age dependent. It has five parameters because there are five parameters in this particular model. Note, the output is similar to that for survival analysis, and the z-statistic is *not* the ratio of the IRR to its SE, but rather the ratio of the log(IRR), log(1.43) to *its* SE.

6.1.4 Model checking

The simplest way to check the model is to compare the observed values and those predicted by the model. The predicted values are obtained by putting the estimated coefficients into equation (6.2). Since the dependent variable is a count we can use a Chi-squared test to compare the observed and predicted values and we obtain $X^2 = 12.13$, d.f. = 4, $P = 0.0164$. This has 4 degrees of freedom (d.f.) because the predicted values are constrained to equal the observed values for the five age groups and one smoking group (the other smoking group constraint follows from the previous age group constraints). Thus six constraints and ten observations yield 4 d.f. There is some evidence that the model does not fit the data. The standardised residuals are defined as $(D - E)/\sqrt{E}$ since the SE of D is $\sqrt{E}$. These are shown in Table 6.1 and we expect most to lie between -2 and $+2$. We can conclude there is little evidence of a systematic lack of fit of the model, except possibly for the non-smokers in the age group 75–84 years, but this is not a large difference.

The only additional term we have available to fit is the smoking × age interaction. This yields a saturated model (i.e. one in which the number of parameters equals the number of data points, see Appendix 2), and its LR Chi-squared is equal to the lack of fit Chi-squared above. Thus there is some evidence that smoking affects coronary risk differently at different ages.

When the observed data vary from the predicted values by more than would be expected by a Poisson distribution we have what is known as *extra-Poisson variation*. This is similar to *extra-Binomial variation* described in Chapter 3. It means that the SEs given by the computer output may not be valid. It may arise because an important covariate is omitted. Another common explanation is when the counts are correlated. This can happen when they refer to counts *within* an individual, such as number of asthma attacks per year, rather than counts within groups of separate individuals. This leads to a random effect model as described in Chapter 5 which, as explained there, will tend to increase our estimate of the SE. Some packages now allow one to fit random effect Poisson models. A particular model that allows for extra variation in the λ_is is known as *negative Binomial regression* and this is available in STATA, for example.

6.1.5 Poisson regression used to estimate relative risks from a 2 × 2 table

Consider again Table 3.1. Rather than the OR, we wish to estimate the *relative risk* of breastfeeding <3 months by profession.

We set up the data as shown in Table 3.1 for the ungrouped analysis, but add an extra column which is an arbitrary constant (say, 1) which is the value e_i in the model. Here we are assuming that all subjects are followed up for the same length of time. We fit a Poisson model but use a "robust SE" estimator to correct the SE because the Poisson assumption is invalid. The output is shown in Table 6.3.

In the output of table 6.3 the relative risk is described as the IRR. As described in Chapter 3 this is estimated as $(36/50)/(30/55) = 1.32$ as shown in Table 6.3. The advantage of this method is we can obtain valid estimates of the CI for the relative risk. With robust SEs the only available test is the Wald test which gives a *P*-value very similar to that given by the Wald test for the logistic regression in Section 3.3.

6.1.6 Poisson regression in action

Campbell *et al.*[5] looked at deaths from asthma over the period 1980–1995 in England and Wales. They used Poisson regression to test whether there was a trend in the deaths over the period, and concluded that, particularly for the

Table 6.3 Using Poisson regression to estimate a relative risk, as a substitute for logistic regression

```
Iteration 0:  log pseudo-likelihood = -96.010221
Iteration 1:  log pseudo-likelihood = -96.010221

Poisson regression                      Number of obs   =      105
                                        Wald chi2(1)    =     3.33
                                        Prob > chi2     =   0.0680
Log pseudo-likelihood = -96.010221      Pseudo R2       =   0.0066
```

y	IRR	Robust Std. Err.	z	P>|z|	[95% Conf. Interval]	
occuptn	1.32	.2008386	1.82	0.068	.9796326	1.778626
one	(exposure)					

age group 15–44, there had been a decline of about 6% (95% CI 5 to 7) per year since 1988, but this downward trend was not evident in the elderly.

6.2 Ordinal regression

When the outcome variable is *ordinal* then the methods described in the earlier chapters are inadequate. One solution would be to dichotomise the data and use logistic regression as discussed in Chapter 3. However, this is inefficient and possibly biased if the point for the dichotomy is chosen by looking at the data. The main model for ordinal regression is known as the *proportional odds* or *cumulative logit model*. It is based on the cumulative response probabilities rather than the category probabilities.

For example consider an ordinal outcome variable Y with k ordered categorical outcomes y_j denoted *by* $j = 1, 2, ..., k$, and let $X_1, ..., X_p$ denote the covariates. The cumulative logit or proportional odds model is

$$\log \text{it}(C_j) = \log_e \left[\frac{C_j}{1 - C_j} \right] = \log_e \left[\frac{\Pr(Y \leq y_j)}{(\Pr(Y > y_j))} \right] = \alpha_i + \beta_1 X_1 + \cdots + \beta_p X_p$$

$$j = 1, 2, ..., k - 1, \tag{6.3}$$

or equivalently as

$$\Pr(Y \leq y_i) = \frac{\exp(\alpha_j + \beta_1 X_1 + \cdots + \beta_p X_p)}{1 + \exp(\alpha_j + \beta_1 X_1 + \cdots + \beta_p X_p)}, \qquad j = 1, 2, ..., k - 1$$

$$\tag{6.4}$$

where $C_j = \Pr(Y \leq y_j)$ is the cumulative probability of being in category j or less (note that for $j = k$; $\Pr(Y \leq y_j \mid X) = 1$). Here we have not used coefficients to indicate individuals to avoid cluttering the notation. Note that we have replaced the intercept term β_0 which would be seen in logistic regression by a set of variables $\alpha_j, j = 1, 2, ..., k - 1$. When there are $k = 2$ categories, this model is identical to equation (3.1), the logistic regression model. When there are more than two categories, we estimate separate intercepts terms for each category except the base category.

The regression coefficients β does not depend on the category i. This implies that the model (6.3) assumes that the relationship between the covariates X and Y is independent of i (the response category). This assumption of identical log ORs across the k categories is known as the *proportional odds assumption*.

The proportional odds model is useful when one believes the dependent variable is continuous, but the values have been grouped for reporting. Alternatively, the variable is measured imperfectly by an instrument with a limited number of values. The division between the boundaries are sometimes known as *cut-points*. The proportional odds model is invariant when the codes for the response Y are reversed (i.e. y_1 recoded as y_k, y_2 recoded as y_{k-1} and so on). Secondly, the proportional odds model is invariant under the collapsibility of adjacent categories of the ordinal response (e.g. y_1 and y_2 combined and y_{k-1} and y_k combined).

Note that count data, described under Poisson regression, could be thought of as ordinal. However, ordinal regression is likely to be inefficient in this case because count data form a ratio scale, and this fact is not utilised in ordinal regression (see Section 1.3).

The interpretation of the model is exactly like that of logistic regression. Continuous and nominal covariates can be included as independent variables.

6.2.1 Interpreting a computer output: ordinal regression

Suppose the length of breastfeeding given in Table 3.1 was measured as <1 month, 1–3 months and $\geqslant 3$ months. Thus, the cut-points are 1 month and 3 months. The data are given in Table 6.4.

The outcome variable is now *ordinal* and it would be sensible to use an analysis that reflected this. In Swinscow and Campbell,[6] the authors showed how this could be done using a non-parametric Mann–Whitney U-test. Ordinal regression is equivalent to the Mann–Whitney test when there is only one independent variable 0/1 in the regression. The advantage of ordinal regression over non-parametric methods is that we get an efficient estimate of a regression coefficient and we can extend the analysis to allow for other confounding variables.

For the analysis we coded printer's wives as 1 and farmer's wives as 0. The dependent variable was coded 1, 2, 3 but in fact many packages will allow any positive whole numbers. The computer analysis is given in Table 6.5. Alas the

Table 6.4 Numbers of wives of printers and farmers who breastfed their babies for <1 month, 1–3 months or for 3 months or more

	<1 month	1–3 months	3 months	Total
Printers' wives	20	16	14	50
Farmers' wives	15	15	25	55
Total	35	31	39	105

Table 6.5 Results of ordinal regression on data in Table 6.4

```
Iteration 0:  log likelihood = -114.89615
Iteration 1:  log likelihood = -113.17681
Iteration 2:  log likelihood = -113.17539

Ordered logit estimates                Number of obs   =      105
                                       LR chi2(1)      =     3.44
                                       Prob > chi2     =   0.0636
Log likelihood = -113.17539            Pseudo R2       =   0.0150

- - - - - - - - - - - - - - - - - - - - - - - - - - - - - - - - - - - -
breast |    Coef.   Std. Err.     z     P>|z|   [95% Conf. Interval]
- - - -+- - - - - - - - - - - - - - - - - - - - - - - - - - - - - - - -
 wives | .671819    .3643271    1.844   0.065   -0.0422491   1.385887
- - - -+- - - - - - - - - - - - - - - - - - - - - - - - - - - - - - - -
 _cut1 | -1.03708    .282662           (Ancillary parameters)
 _cut2 | .2156908   .2632804
- - - - - - - - - - - - - - - - - - - - - - - - - - - - - - - - - - - -
```

computer output does not give the ORs and so we have to compute them ourselves. Thus, the OR is $\exp(0.672) = 1.96$ with 95% CI as $\exp(-0.042)$ to $\exp(1.386)$ which is 0.96 to 4.0. This contrasts with the OR of 2.14 (95% CI 0.95 to 4.84) that we obtained in Table 3.2 when we had only two categories for the dependent variable. The interpretation is that after 1 month, and after 3 months, a printer's wife has twice the odds of being in the same breastfeeding category *or lower* as a farmer's wife.

The LR Chi-square has 1 d.f., corresponding to the single term in the model. The *P*-value associated with it, 0.0636, agrees closely with the Wald *P*-value of 0.065. The two intercepts are labelled in the output _cut1 and _cut2. They are known as *ancillary parameters*, meaning that they are extra parameters introduced to fit the model, but not part of the inferential study. Thus no significance levels are attached to them.

Useful discussions of the proportional odds model and other models for ordinal data have been given by Armstrong and Sloan,[7] and Ananth and Kleinbaum.[8] Other models include the *continuation ratio model*. Armstrong and Sloan[7] conclude that the gain in efficiency using a proportional odds model as opposed to logistic regression is often not great, especially when the majority of the observations fall in one category. The strategy of dichotomising an ordinal variable and using logistic regression has much to recommend it in terms of simplicity and ease of interpretation, unless the coefficient of the main predictor variable is close to borderline significance. However, it is very important that the point of dichotomy is chosen *a priori* and not after having inspected several choices and choosing the one that closest conforms to our prejudices.

6.2.2 Model checking

Tests are available for proportional odds but these tests lack power. Also the model is robust to mild departures from the assumption of proportional odds. A crude test would be to examine the ORs associated with each cutpoint. If they are all greater than unity, or all less than unity, then a proportional odds model will suffice.

From Table 6.3 we find the odds are:

$<$1 month vs $\geqslant$1 month $\qquad\qquad$ $<$3 months vs $\geqslant$3 months

$$OR = \frac{20 \times 40}{15 \times 30} = 1.78 \qquad\qquad OR = \frac{36 \times 25}{30 \times 14} = 2.14$$

These ORs are quite close to each other and we can see that the observed OR of 1.96 from the proportional odds model is midway between the two. Thus we have no reason to reject the proportional odds model. Experience has shown that provided the odds do not actually change direction (i.e. the second odds being the other side of unity to the first one) then the proportional odds model is pretty robust.[9]

Model testing is much more complicated when there is more than one input variable and some of them are continuous, and specialist help should be sought.

6.2.3 Ordinal regression in action

Hotopf *et al.*[10] looked at the relationship between chronic childhood abdominal pain as measured on three consecutive surveys at ages 7, 11 and 15 years and adult psychiatric disorders at the age of 36 years, in a cohort of 3637 individuals. A 7 point index of psychiatric disorder (the "index of definition") was measured as an outcome variable. This is an ordinal scale. It was found that the binary predictor (causal) variable, pain on all three surveys, was associated with an OR of 2.72 (95% CI 1.65 to 4.49) when potential confounders sex, father's social class, marital status at age 36 years and educational status were included in the model. Thus the authors conclude that children with abdominal pain are more likely to present psychiatric problems in later life. The usual cutoff for the index of definition is 5, but use of the whole scale uses more information and so gives more precise estimates.

6.3 Time series regression

Time series regression is concerned with the situation in which the dependent and independent variables are measured over time. Usually there is only a single series with one dependent variable and a number of independent variables, unlike repeated measures when there may be several series of data.

The potential for confounding in time series regression is very high – many variables either simply increase or decrease over time, and so will be correlated over time.[11] In addition, many epidemiological variables are seasonal, and this variation would be present even if the factors were not causally related. It is important that seasonality and trends are properly accounted for. Simply because the outcome variable is seasonal, it is impossible to ascribe causality because of seasonality of the predictor variable. For example, sudden infant deaths are higher in winter than in summer, but this does not imply that temperature is a causal factor; there are many other factors that might affect the result such as reduced daylight, or presence of viruses. However, if an unexpectedly cold winter is associated with an increase in sudden infant deaths, or very cold days are consistently followed after a short time by rises in the daily sudden infant death rate, then causality may possibly be inferred.

Often when confounding factors are correctly accounted for, the serial correlation of the residuals disappears; they appear serially correlated because of the association with a time dependent predictor variable, and so conditional on this variable the residuals are independent. This is particularly likely for mortality data, where, except in epidemics, the individual deaths are unrelated. Thus, one can often use conventional regression methods followed by a check for the serial correlation of the residuals and need only proceed further if there is clear evidence of a lack of independence.

If the inclusion of known or potential confounders fails to remove the serial correlation of the residuals, then it is known that ordinary least squares does not provide valid estimates of the SEs of the parameters.

6.3.1 The model

For a continuous outcome, suppose the model is

$$y_i = \beta_0 + \beta_1 X_{t1} + \cdots + \beta_p X_{tp} + \nu_t, t = 1, \ldots, n. \qquad (6.5)$$

The main difference from equation (2.1) is that we now index time t rather than individuals. It is important to distinguish time points because whereas two individuals with the same covariates are interchangeable, you cannot swap, say Saturday with Sunday and expect the same results! We denote the error term by ν_t and we assume that $\nu_t = \varepsilon_t - \alpha \nu_{t-1}$ where the ε_t are assumed independent Normally distributed variables with mean 0 and variance σ^2 and α is a constant between -1 and $+1$. The error term is known as an *autoregressive process (of order 1)*. This model implies that the data are correlated in time, known as *serial correlation*. The effect of ignoring serial correlation is to provide artificially low estimates of the SE of the regression coefficients and thus to imply significance more often than the significance level would suggest, under the null hypothesis of no association.

6.3.2 Estimation using correlated residuals

Given the above model, and assuming α is known, we can use a method of generalised least squares known as the *Cochrane–Orcutt procedure*.[12]

For simplicity assume one independent variable and write $y_t^* = y_t - \alpha y_{t-1}$ and $x_t^* = X_t - \alpha X_{t-1}$. We can then obtain an estimate of β using ordinary least squares on y_t^* and x_t^*. However, since α will not usually be known it can be estimated from the ordinary least squares residuals e_t by

$$a = \frac{\sum_{t=2}^{n} e_t e_{t-1}}{\sum_{t=2}^{n} e_{t-1}^2}.$$

This leads to an iterative procedure in which we can construct a new set of transformed variables and thus a new set of regression estimates and so on until convergence. The iterative Cochrane–Orcutt procedure can be interpreted as a stepwise algorithm for computing maximum likelihood estimators of α and β where the initial observation y_1 is regarded as fixed. If the residuals are assumed to be Normally distributed then full maximum likelihood methods are available, which estimate α and β simultaneously. This can be generalised to higher order autoregressive models and fitted in a number of computer packages, in particular SAS. However, caution is advised in using this method when the autocorrelations are high, and it is worth making the point that an autoregressive error model "should not be used as a nostrum for models that simply do not fit".[13]

There are more modern methods which do not assume the first point is fixed, but if the data set is long (say, >50 points) then the improvement is minimal. These models can be generalised to outcomes which are counts but this is beyond the scope of this book and for further details see Campbell.[14]

6.3.3 Interpreting a computer output: time series regression

Suppose that the data on deadspace and height in Table 2.1 in fact referred to one individual followed up over time. Then the regression of deadspace against height is given in Table 6.6 using Cochrane–Orcutt regression. This method loses the first observation, and so the regression coefficient is not strictly comparable with that in Figure 2.1. Note that the output gives the number of observations as 14, not 15. Note also that the SE, 0.214 obtained here, is much larger than the 0.180 obtained when all the points are assumed to be independent. The estimate of α, the autocorrelation coefficient is denoted rho in the printout and is quite small at 0.046 (as might be expected since the data are not, in fact, autocorrelated). However, the program does not give a P-value for rho.

Table 6.6 Results of Cochrane–Orcutt regression on data in Table 2.1 assuming points all belong to one individual over time

```
Iteration 0:   rho = 0.0000
Iteration 1:   rho = 0.0432
Iteration 2:   rho = 0.0462
Iteration 3:   rho = 0.0463
Iteration 4:   rho = 0.0463
Iteration 5:   rho = 0.0463
```

Cochrane–Orcutt AR(1) regression -- iterated estimates

Source	SS	df	MS		Number of obs	=	14
					F(1, 12)	=	29.29
Model	4841.31415	1	4841.31415		Prob > F	=	0.0002
Residual	1983.76032	12	165.31336		R-squared	=	0.7093
					Adj R-squared	=	0.6851
Total	6825.07447	13	525.005728		Root MSE	=	12.857

Deadspce	Coef.	Std. Err.	t	P>|t|	[95% Conf. Interval]	
Height	1.160173	.2143853	5.412	0.000	.6930675	1.627279
_cons	-102.1168	31.78251	-3.213	0.007	-171.3649	-32.86861
rho	.0463493					

```
Durbin-Watson statistic (original)      1.834073
Durbin-Watson statistic (transformed)   1.901575
```

6.4 Reporting Poisson, ordinal or time series regression in the literature

- If the dependent variable is a count then Poisson regression may be the required model. Give evidence that the model is a reasonable fit to the data by quoting the goodness-of-fit Chi-squared. Test for covariate interaction or allow for extra-Poisson variation if the model is not a good fit.
- If the dependent variable is ordinal, then ordinal regression *may* be useful. However, if the ordinal variable has a large number of categories (say, >7) then linear regression may be suitable. Give evidence that the proportional odds model is a reasonable one, perhaps by quoting the ORs associated with each cut-point for the main independent variable. If proportional odds assumption is unlikely, then dichotomise the dependent variable and use logistic regression. *Do not* choose the point for dichotomy by choosing the one that gives the most significant value for the primary independent variable!
- When the data form a time series, look for evidence that the residuals in the model are serially correlated. If they are, then include a term in the model to allow for serial correlation.

6.5   Reading about the results of Poisson, ordinal or time series regression in the literature

- As usual, look for evidence that the model is reasonable
- In Poisson regression, are the counts independent? If not, should over-dispersion be considered?
- If ordinal regression has been used, how has the result been interpreted?
- A common error in time series regression is to ignore serial correlation. This may not invalidate the analysis, but it is worth asking whether it might. Another common feature is to only use a first order autoregression to allow for serial correlation, but it may be worth asking whether this is sufficient and whether a higher order autoregression would be better.

EXERCISES

1 Stene et al.[15] looked at all live births in Norway from 1974 to 1998 and found 1828 children diagnosed with diabetes between 1989 and 1998. They fitted a Poisson regression model to the number of incident cases (D_j) and the person-time under observation (T_j) in each exposure category j. All confounders, such as maternal age and period of birth, were categorised. They investigated the relationship between birth weight and incidence of Type 1 diabetes and found an almost linear relationship. They tested for interactions between birth weight and different categories of gestational age and found no interaction. In terms of model fit, they showed a graph of incidence of diabetes vs birth weight and stated that they tested for interactions.

   (i) Why were the potential confounders categorised?

   (ii) If a graph of incidence vs birth weight shows a straight line, is this reflected by the model?

   (iii) What other tests of the model might one employ?

   (iv) What other statistical model might be appropriate here?

2 Wight et al.[16] carried out a survey of 3665 boys and 3730 girls aged under 16 years in Scotland. The main question was about sexual intercourse and 661 boys and 576 girls admitted to having had sex. The main outcome was whether their first time was "at the right age" (55% girls, 68% boys), "too early" (32% girls, 27% boys) or "should not have happened" (13% girls, 5% boys). The authors were interested in the effect of gender on this outcome, and whether this was affected by social class and parenting style.

What type of variable is the outcome variable? Describe what type of model to fit to this outcome, how it might be better than logistic regression, and how a multivariate model could be used to adjust for social class and parenting style. Discuss the assumptions for the model and give an informal check for the effect of gender on the outcome.

References

1. McNeil D. *Epidemiological Research Methods*. Chichester: John Wiley, 1996.
2. Breslow NE, Day NE. *Statistical Methods in Cancer Research: Vol II — The Design and Analysis of Cohort Studies*. Lyon: IARC, 1987.
3. Zou G. A modified Poisson regression approach to prospective studies with binary data. *Am J Epidemiol* 2004; **159:** 702–6.
4. Doll R, Hill AB. Mortality of British doctors in relation to smoking: observations on coronary thrombosis. *Natl Cancer Inst Monog* 1996; **19:** 205–68.
5. Campbell MJ, Cogman GR, Holgate ST, Johnston SL. Age specific trends in asthma mortality in England and Wales 1983–1995: results of an observational study. *Br Med J* 1997; **314:** 1439–41.
6. Swinscow TDV, Campbell MJ. *Statistics at Square One*, 10th edn. London: BMJ Books, 2002.
7. Armstrong BG, Sloan M. Ordinal regression models for epidemiologic data. *Am J Epidemiol* 1989; **129:** 191–204.
8. Ananth CV, Kleinbaum DG. Regression models for ordinal responses: a review of methods and applications. *Int J Epidemiol* 1997; **26:** 1323–33.
9. Lall R, Walters SJ, Campbell MJ, Morgan K and MRC CFAS. A review of ordinal regression models applied on Health Related Quality of Life Assessments. *Stat Meth Med Res* 2002; **11:** 49–66.
10. Hotopf M, Carr S, Magou R, Wadsworth M, Wessely S. Why do children have chronic abdominal pain and what happens to them when they grow up? Population based cohort study. *Br Med J* 1998; **316:** 1196–200.
11. Yule GU. Why do we sometimes get nonsense correlations between time series? A study in sampling and the nature of time-series. *J Roy Statist Soc* 1926; **89:** 187–227.
12. Cochrane D, Orcutt GH. Application of least squares regression to relationships containing autocorrelated error terms. *J Am Statist Assoc* 1949; **44:** 32–61.
13. SAS Institute Inc. *SAS/ETS User's Guide Version 5 Edition*. Cary, NC: SAS Institute, 1984; 192.
14. Campbell MJ. Time series regression. In: Armitage P, Colton T, eds. *Encyclopaedia of Biostatistics*. Chichester: John Wiley, 1997: 4536–8.
15. Stene LC, Magnus P, Lie RT, Søvik O, Joner G, *et al.* Birth weight and childhood onset type I diabetes: population based cohort study. *Br Med J* 2001; **322:** 889–92.
16. Wight D, Henderson M, Raab G, Abraham C, Buston K, *et al.* Extent of regretted sexual intercourse among young teenagers in Scotland: a cross-sectional survey. *Br Med J* 2000; **320:** 1243–4.

Appendix 1 **Exponentials and logarithms**

A1.1 Logarithms

It is simple to understand raising a quantity to a power, so that $y = x^2$ is equivalent to $y = x \times x$. This can be generalised *to* $y = x^n$ for arbitrary n so $y = x \times x \times \ldots \times x$ n times.

A simple result is that

$$x^n \times x^m = x^{n+m} \tag{A1.1}$$

for arbitrary n and m. Thus, for example $3^2 \times 3^4 = 3^6 = 729$. It can be shown that this holds for *any* values of m and n, not just whole numbers.

We define $x^0 = 1$, because $x^n = x^{0+n} = x^0 \times x^n = 1 \times x^n$.

A useful extension of the concept of powers is to let n take fractional or negative values. Thus $y = x^{0.5}$ can be shown to be equivalent to $y = \sqrt{x}$, because $x^{0.5} \times x^{0.5} = x^{0.5+0.5} = x^1 = x$ and also $\sqrt{x} \times \sqrt{x} = x$.

Also x^{-1} can be shown equivalent to $1/x$, because $x \times x^{-1} = x^{1-1} = x^0 = 1$.

If $y = x^n$, then the definition of a logarithm of y to the base x is the power that x has to be raised to get y. This is written $n = \log_x(y)$ or "n equals log to the base x of y".

Suppose $y = x^n$ and $z = x^m$. It can be shown from equation (A1.1) that

$$\log_x(y \times z) = n + m = \log_x(y) + \log_x(z).$$

Thus, when we multiply two numbers we add their logs. This was the basis of the original use of logarithms in that they enabled a transformation whereby arithmetic using multiplications could be done using additions, which are much easier to do by hand. In Appendix 2 we need an equivalent result, namely that

$$\log_x\left(\frac{y}{z}\right) = \log_x(y) - \log_x(z).$$

In other words, when we log transform the ratio of two numbers we subtract the logs of the two numbers.

The two most common bases are 10, and a strange quantity e = 2.718...,
where the dots indicate that the decimals go on indefinitely. This number has
the useful property that the slope of the curve $y = e^x$ at any point (x, y) is just y,
whereas for all other bases the slope is proportional to y but not exactly equal to
it. The formula $y = e^x$ is often written $y = \exp(x)$. The logarithms to base e and
10 are often denoted ln and log respectively on calculators, and the former is
often called the *natural logarithm*. In this book all logarithms are natural, that
is to base e. We can get from one base to the other by noting that $\log_{10}(y) = \log_e(y) \times \log_{10}(e)$. To find the value of e on a calculator enter 1 and press *exp*.
$\log_{10}(e)$ is a constant equal to 0.4343. Thus $\log_{10} y = 0.4343 \times \log_e(y)$.

Try this on a calculator. Put in any positive number and press *ln* and then
exp. You will get back to the original number because $\exp[\ln(x)] = x$.

Note it follows from the definition that for any $x > 0$, $\log_x(1) = 0$. Try this
on a calculator for log(1) and ln(1).

In this book exponentials and logarithms feature in a number of places. It is
much easier to model data as additive terms in a linear predictor, and yet often
terms, such as risk, behave multiplicatively, as discussed in Chapter 3. Taking
logs transforms the model from a multiplicative one to an additive one.
Logarithms are also commonly used to transform variables which have a posi-
tively skewed distribution, because it has been found that this often makes their
distribution closer to a Normal distribution. This, of course, will not work if
the variable can be 0 or negative. A graph of $\log_e(x)$ vs x is shown in Figure
A1.1. The line does not plateau, but the rate of increase gets small as x increases.

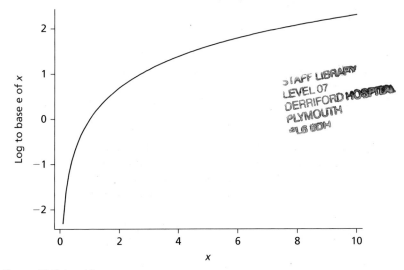

Figure A1.1 $\log_e(x)$ vs x.

Appendix 2 **Maximum likelihood and significance tests**

Summary

This appendix gives a brief introduction to the use of *maximum likelihood*, which was the method used to fit the models in the earlier chapters. We describe the *Wald test* and the *likelihood ratio (LR) test* and link the latter to the *deviance*. Further details are given in Clayton and Hills.[1]

A2.1 Binomial models and likelihood

A *model* is a structure for describing data and consists of two parts. The first part describes how the explanatory variables are combined in a linear fashion to give a linear predictor. This is then transformed by a function known as a *link* function to give predicted or fitted values of the outcome variable for an individual. The second part of the model describes the probability distribution of the outcome variable about the predicted value.

Perhaps the simplest model is the Binomial model. An event happens with a probability π. Suppose the event is the probability of giving birth to a boy and suppose we had 5 expectant mothers who subsequently gave birth to 2 boys and 3 girls. The boys were born to mothers numbered 1 and 3. If π is the probability of a boy the probability of this sequence of events occurring is $\pi \times (1 - \pi) \times \pi \times (1 - \pi) \times (1 - \pi)$. If the mothers had different characteristics, say their age, we might wish to distinguish them and write the probability of a boy for mother i as π_i and the probability of a girl as $(1 - \pi_i)$ and the probability of the sequence as $\pi_1 \times (1 - \pi_2) \times \pi_3 \times (1 - \pi_4) \times (1 - \pi_5)$. For philosophical and semantic reasons this probability is termed the *likelihood* (in normal parlance likelihood and probability are synonyms) for this particular sequence of events and in this case is written $L(\pi)$. The likelihood is the probability of the data, *given* the model.

The process of *maximum likelihood* is to choose values of the πs which maximise the likelihood. In Chapter 3, we discussed models for the πs which are functions of the subject characteristics. For simplicity, here we will consider two extreme cases: (i) the πs are all the same so we have no information to distinguish individuals, (ii) each π is determined by the data, and we can choose each π by whether the outcome is a boy or a girl. In the latter case we can simply choose $\pi_1 = \pi_3 = 1$ and $\pi_2 = \pi_4 = \pi_5 = 0$. This is a *saturated model*, so called because we saturate the model with parameters, and the maximum number possible is to have as many parameters as there are data points (or strictly *degrees of freedom* (*d.f.*)). In this case

$$L(\pi) = 1 \times (1 - 0) \times 1 \times (1 - 0) \times (1 - 0) = 1.$$

If the πs are all the same, then $L(\pi) = \pi \times (1 - \pi) \times \pi \times (1 - \pi) \times (1 - \pi) = \pi^2(1 - \pi)^3$. In general if there were D boys in N births then $L(\pi) = \pi^D(1 - \pi)^{N-D}$. The likelihood, for any particular values of π is a very small number, and it is more convenient to use the natural logarithm of the likelihood instead of the likelihood itself. In this way

$$\log_e[L(\pi)] = D\log_e(\pi) + (N - D)\log_e(1 - \pi). \tag{A2.1}$$

It is simple to show that the value of π that maximises the likelihood is the same value that maximises the log-likelihood.

In the expression (A2.1), the data provide N and D and the statistical problem is to see how $\log[L(\pi)]$ varies as we vary π, and to choose the value of π that most closely agrees with the data. This is the value of π that maximises $\log[L(\pi)]$. A graph of the log-likelihood for the data above (2 boys and 3 girls) is given in Figure A2.1.

The maximum occurs at $\pi = 0.4$, which is what one might have guessed. The value at the maximum is given by

$$[L(\pi_{max})] = 2\log_e(0.4) + 3\log_e(1 - 0.4) = -3.3651.$$

The graph, however, is very flat, implying that the maximum is not well estimated. This is because we have very little information with only five observations.

For reasons to be discussed later, the equation for the likelihood is often scaled by the value of the likelihood at the maximum, to give the likelihood ratio, LR(π):

$$LR(\pi) = \frac{L(\pi)}{L(\pi_{max})} \qquad 0 < \pi < 1.$$

When we take logs (as described in Appendix 1) this becomes

$$\log_e[LR(\pi)] = \log_e[L(\pi)] - \log_e[L(\pi_{max})].$$

Again the maximum occurs when $\pi = 0.4$, but in this case the maximum value is 0.

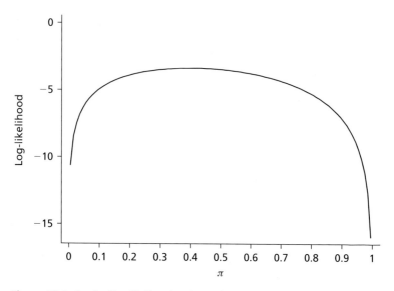

Figure A2.1 Graph of log-likelihood against π, for a Binomial model with $D = 2$ and $N = 5$.

A2.2 Poisson model

The Poisson model, discussed in Chapter 6, is useful when the number of subjects N is large and the probability of an event, π, is small. Then the expected number of events $\lambda = N\pi$ is moderate.

In this case the likelihood for an observed count D is $L(\lambda) = e^{-\lambda}\lambda^D$ and the log-likelihood is

$$\log_e[L(\lambda)] = D\log_e(\lambda) - \lambda.$$

A2.3 Normal model

The probability distribution for a variable Y which has a Normal distribution with mean μ and standard deviation σ is given by

$$\frac{0.3989}{\sigma}\exp\left[\frac{-1}{2}\left(\frac{y-\mu}{\sigma}\right)^2\right].$$

This value changes with differing μ and differing σ. If σ is known (and thus fixed), then this likelihood is simply equal to the above probability but now does not vary with σ and is a function of μ only, which we denote $L(\mu)$.

For a series of observations $y_1, y_2, \ldots, y_n$ the log-likelihood is

$$\log_e[L(\mu)] = k - \frac{1}{2\sigma^2}\sum_{i=1}^{n}(y_i - \mu)^2$$

where k is a constant.

A saturated model will have n parameters $\mu_1 = y_1$, $\mu_2 = y_2$, etc. and $\log_e[L(\mu_1, \ldots, \mu_n)] = k$.

Thus the log LR is

$$\log_e[L(\mu)] = -\frac{1}{2\sigma^2}\sum_{i=1}^{n}(y_i - \mu)^2. \qquad (A2.2)$$

It is easy to show that to *maximise* the log LR we have to minimise the sum on the right-hand side of (A2.2), because the quantity on the right is negative and small absolute negative values are bigger than large absolute negative values (-1 is bigger than -2). Thus, we have to choose a value to minimise the sum of squares of the observations from μ. This is the *principle of least squares* described in Chapter 2, and we can see it is equivalent to maximising the likelihood.

The maximum value occurs when

$$\hat{\mu} = \sum_{i=1}^{n}\frac{y_i}{n} = \bar{y}.$$

Suppose we know that adult male height has a Normal distribution. We do not know the mean μ, but we do know the standard deviation to be 15 cm. Imagine 10 men selected at random from this population with an average height of 175 cm. The mean of a set of n observations from a Normal distribution with mean μ and variance σ^2 is itself Normally distributed with mean μ and variance σ^2/n.

Then the log LR for these data against a theoretical value μ is

$$\log_e[LR(\mu)] = -\frac{n}{2\sigma^2}(\bar{y} - \mu)^2.$$

For our data this is given by

$$\log_e[LR(\mu)] = -\frac{10}{2}\frac{(175 - \mu)^2}{15}. \qquad (A2.3)$$

This is shown in Figure A2.2 for different values of μ. Curves with this form are called *quadratic*.

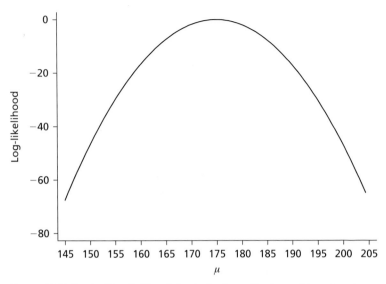

Figure A2.2 Graph of log-likelihood of a single observation from a Normal model.

A2.4 Hypothesis testing: LR test

Suppose we wished to test the hypothesis that the population from which these men were drawn had a mean height of 170 cm.

Before we can calculate the hypothesis test, we must first use a most useful result for the Normal distribution. The result is that under the Normal distribution:

$$-2 \times (\text{observed log LR})$$

is distributed as a Chi-squared distribution with 1 d.f.

Suppose μ_0 was 170. Then $-2 \times \log \text{LR}$ is $2 \times 10 \times (175 - 170)^2/(2 \times 15) = 16.7$. This is well in excess of the 1% value of a Chi-squared distribution with 1 d.f. of 6.63 and so, with our observation of a mean of 175 cm we can reject the null hypothesis that $\mu_0 = 170$.

For non-Normal data the result that $-2 \times (\text{observed log LR})$ is distributed as a Chi-squared distribution is approximately true, and the distribution gets closer to a Chi-squared distribution as the sample size increases. Returning to our birth data, suppose our null hypothesis was $\pi_0 = 0.5$, that is, boys and girls are equally likely. The log-likelihood is $2 \times \log(0.5) + 3 \times \log(0.5) = -3.4657$ and the corresponding log LR is $-3.4657 - (-3.3651) = -0.1006$.

We have $-2 \times \log \text{LR} = 0.20$, which is much less than the tabulated Chi-squared value of 3.84 and so we cannot reject the null hypothesis. Here the approximation to a Chi-squared distribution is likely to be poor because of the small sample size. Intuitively we can see that, because the curve in Figure A2.1 is far from quadratic. However, as the sample size increases it will become closer to a quadratic curve.

The log-likelihood is a measure of *goodness-of-fit* of a model. The greater the log-likelihood the better the fit. Since the absolute value of the log-likelihood is not itself of interest, it is often reported as a log LR compared to some other model. Many computer programs report the *deviance*, which is minus twice the log LR of the model being fitted and a saturated model which includes the maximum number of terms in the model (say as many terms as there are observations). For the birth data above, the saturated model had five parameters, the likelihood was 1 and the log-likelihood 0, and so the deviance in this case is the same as the log-likelihood times minus two. The deviance has d.f. equal to the difference between the number of parameters in the model and the number of parameters in the saturated model.

The deviance is really a measure of badness-of-fit, not goodness-of-fit; a large deviance indicates a bad fit. If one model is a subset of another, in that the larger model contains the parameters of the smaller, then they can be compared using the differences in their deviances. The change in deviance is minus twice the log LR for the two models because the log-likelihood for the saturated model occurs in both deviances and cancels. The d.f. for this test are found by subtracting the d.f. for the two deviances.

A2.5 Wald test

When the data are not Normally distributed, the shape of the log LR is no longer quadratic. However, as can be seen from Figure A2.1, it is often approximately so, especially for large samples and there can be advantages in terms of simplicity to using the best quadratic approximation rather than the true likelihood.

Consider a likelihood for a parameter θ of a probability model and let M be the most likely value of θ. A simple quadratic expression is

$$\log[\mathrm{LR}(\theta)] = -\frac{1}{2}\left(\frac{M-\theta}{S}\right)^2.$$

This is known as the Wald LR and has a maximum value of 0 when $M = \theta$, and can be used to approximate the true log LR. The parameter S is known as the standard error (SE) of the estimate and is used to scale the curve. Small values give sharp peaks of the quadratic curve and large values give flatter peaks. S is chosen to give the closest approximation to the true likelihood *in the region of its most likely value*.

For the binary data given above, with D events out of N the values of M and S are

$$M = \frac{D}{N}$$

and

$$S = \sqrt{\frac{M(1 - M)}{N}}.$$

For $D = 2$ and $N = 5$ we get $M = 0.4$ and $S = 0.22$.

Under the null hypothesis of $\theta = 0.5$, we find that for the Wald LR $-2 \times \log_e$ LR is

$$\left(\frac{0.4 - 0.5}{0.22}\right)^2 = 0.21.$$

This is close to the log LR value of 0.20 and once again is not statistically significant. This test is commonly used because computer programs obligingly produce estimates of SEs of parameters. This is equivalent to the z-test described in Swinscow and Campbell[2] of $b/\mathrm{SE}(b)$.

A2.6   Score test

The score test features less often and so we will not describe it in detail. It is based on the gradient of the log LR curve at the null hypothesis. The gradient is often denoted by U and known as the score, evaluated at the null value of the parameter θ_0. Since the slope of a curve at its maximum is 0, if the null hypothesis coincides with the most likely value, then clearly $U = 0$. The score test is based on the fact that under the null hypothesis U^2/V is approximately distributed as a Chi-squared distribution with 1 d.f., where V is an estimate of the square of the SE of the score.

A2.7   Which method to choose?

For non-Normal data, the methods given above are all approximations. The advantage of the log LR method is that it gives the same P-value even if the parameter is transformed (such as by taking logarithms), and so is the generally preferred method. If the three methods give seriously different results, it means that the quadratic approximations are not sufficiently close to the true log-likelihood curve in the region going from the null value to the most likely value. This is particularly true if the null value and the most likely value are very far apart, and in this case the choice of the statistical method is most unlikely to affect our scientific conclusions. The Wald test can be improved by a suitable transformation. For example, in a model which includes an odds ratio (OR), reformulating the model for a log OR will improve the quadratic approximation, which is another reason why the log OR is a suitable model in Chapter 3.

All three methods can be generalised to test a number of parameters simultaneously. However, if one uses a computer program to fit two models, one of which is a subset of the other, then the log-likelihood or the deviance is usually given for each model from which one can derive the log LR for the two models. If the larger model contains two or more parameters more than the smaller model, then the log LR test of whether the enhanced model significantly improves the fit of the data is a test of all the extra parameters simultaneously.

The parameter estimates and their SEs are given for each term in a model in a computer output, from which the Wald tests can be derived for each parameter. Thus the simple Wald test tests each parameter separately, not simultaneously with the others. Examples are given in the relevant chapters.

A2.8 Confidence intervals

The conventional approach to confidence intervals (CIs) is to use the Wald approach. Thus an approximate 95% CI of a population parameter, for which we have an estimate and a SE is given by an estimate plus $2 \times$ SE to estimate minus $2 \times$ SE. Thus for the birth data an approximate 95% CI is given by $0.6 - 2 \times 0.22$ to $0.6 + 2 \times 0.22 = 0.16$ to 1.04. This immediately shows how poor the approximation is because we cannot have a proportion >1. (for better approximations see Altman et al.)[3] As in the case of the Wald test, the

---

EXAMPLE: DERIVE THE LOG-LIKELIHOODS GIVEN IN TABLE 3.2

Under the null hypothesis the best estimate of the probability of breast feeding for <3 months is $66/105 = 0.629$. From equation (A2.1) we have $D = 66$ and $N = 105$ and so $\log[L(\pi)] = 66 \ln(0.629) + 39 \ln(0.371) = -69.2697$. Under the alternative hypothesis we have $D_1 = 36$, $N_1 = 50$ and $\pi_1 = 36/50 = 0.72$ and $D_2 = 30$, $N_2 = 55$ and $\pi_2 = 0.5454$. Thus $\log[L(\pi_1, \pi_2)] = 36 \ln(0.72) + 14 \ln(0.28) + 30 \ln(0.5454) + 25 \ln(0.4546) = -67.5432$ as given in Table 3.2.

approximation is improved by a suitable transformation, which is why in Chapter 3 we worked on the log OR, rather than the OR itself. However it is possible to calculate CIs directly from the likelihood which do not require a transformation, and these are occasionally given in the literature. For further details see Clayton and Hills.[1]

References

1. Clayton D, Hills M. *Statistical Models in Epidemiology*. Oxford: OUP, 1993.
2. Swinscow TDV, Campbell MJ. *Statistics at Square One*, 10th edn. London: BMJ Books, 2000.
3. Altman DG, Machin D, Bryant TN, Gardner MJ, eds. *Statistics with Confidence*, 2nd edn. London: BMJ Books, 2000.

Appendix 3 **Bootstrapping and variance robust standard errors**

Bootstrapping is a computer intensive method for estimating parameters and confidence intervals (CIs) for models that requires fewer assumptions about the distribution of the data than the parametric methods discussed so far. It is becoming much easier to carry out and is available on most modern computer packages.

All the models so far discussed require assumptions concerning the sampling distribution of the estimate of interest. If the sample size is large and we wish to estimate a CI for a mean, then the underlying population distribution is not important because the central limit theorem will ensure that the sampling distribution is approximately Normal. However, if the sample size is small we can only assume a t-distribution if the underlying population distribution can be assumed Normal. If this is not the case then the interval cannot be expected to cover the population value with the specified confidence. However, we have information on the distribution of the population from the distribution of the sample data. So-called "bootstrap" estimates (from the expression "pulling oneself up by one's bootstraps") utilise this information, by making repeated random samples of the same size as the original sample from the data, with replacement using a computer. Suitable references are Efron and Tibshirani,[1] and Davison and Hinckley.[2]

We seek to mimic in an appropriate manner the way the sample is collected from the population in the bootstrap samples from the observed data. The "with replacement" means that any observation can be sampled more than once. It is important because sampling without replacement would simply give a random permutation of the original data, with many statistics such as the mean being exactly the same. It turns out that "with replacement" is the best way to do this if the observations are independent; if they are not then other methods, beyond the scope of this article, are needed. The standard error (SE) or CI is estimated from the variability of the statistic derived from the bootstrap samples. The point about the bootstrap is that it produces a variety of values, whose variability reflects the SE which would be obtained if samples were repeatedly taken from the whole population.

Suppose we wish to calculate a 95% CI for a mean. We take a random sample of the data, of the same size as the original sample, and calculate the mean of the data in this random sample. We do this repeatedly, say 999 times. We now have 999 means. If these are ordered in increasing value a bootstrap 95% CI for the mean would be from the 25th to the 975th values. This is known as the *percentile method* and although it is an obvious choice, it is not the best method of bootstrapping because it can have a bias, which one can estimate and correct for. This leads to methods, such as the *bias-corrected method* and the *bias-corrected and accelerated (BCa) method*, the latter being the preferred option. When analysis involves an explicit model we can use the "parametric bootstrap". In this case, the model is fitted and the estimated coefficients, the fitted values and residuals stored. The residuals are then randomly sampled with replacement, and then these bootstrapped residuals are added to the fitted values to give a new dependent variable. The model is then estimated again, and the procedure repeated. The sequence of estimated coefficients gives us the distribution from which we can derive the bootstrap statistics.

Using the methods above, valid bootstrap *P*-values and CIs can be constructed for all common estimators, such as a proportion, a median, or a difference in means provided the data are independent and come from the same population.

The number of samples required depends on the type of estimator: 50–200 are adequate for a CI for a mean, but 1000 are required for a CI of, say, the 2.5% or 97.5% centiles.

EXAMPLE

Consider the beta-endorphin concentrations from 11 runners described by Dale *et al.*[3] and also described in Altman *et al.* (Chapter 13).[4] To calculate a 95% CI for the median using a bootstrap we proceed as follows:

Beta-endorphin concentrations in pmol/l		Median
Original sample:	66, 71.2, 83.0, 83.6, 101, 107.6, 122, 143, 160, 177, 414	107.6
Bootstrap 1:	143, 107.6, 414, 160, 101, 177, 107.6, 160, 160, 160, 101	160
Bootstrap 2:	122, 414, 101, 83.6, 143, 107.6, 101, 143, 143, 143, 107.6	122
Bootstrap 3:	122, 414, 160, 177, 101, 107.6, 83.6, 177, 177, 107.6, 107.6	122
etc. 999 times		

The medians are then ordered by increasing value. The 25th and the 975th values out of 1000 give the percentile estimates of the 95% CI. Using 999 replications we find that the BCa method gives a 95% bootstrap CI 71.2 to 143.0 pmol/l. This contrasts with 71.2 to 177 pmol/l using standard methods given in Chapter 5 of Altman *et al.*[4] This suggests that the lower limit for the standard method is probably about right but the upper limit may be too high.

When the standard and the bootstrap methods agree, we can be more confident about the inference we are making and this is an important use of the bootstrap. When they disagree more caution is needed, but the relatively simple assumptions required by the bootstrap method for validity mean that in general it is to be preferred.

It may seem that the best estimator of the median for the population is the median of the bootstrap estimates, but this turns out not to be the case, and one should quote the sample median as the best estimate of the population median.

The main advantage of the bootstrap is that it frees the investigator from making inappropriate assumptions about the distribution of an estimator in order to make inferences. A particular advantage is that it is available when the formula cannot be derived and it may provide better estimates when the formulae are only approximate.

The so-called "naïve" bootstrap makes the assumption that the sample is an unbiased simple random sample from the study population. More complex sampling schemes, such as stratified random sampling may not be reflected by this, and more complex bootstrapping schemes may be required. Naïve bootstrapping may not be successful in very small samples (say, <9 observations), which are less likely to be representative of the study population. "In very small samples even a badly fitting parametric analysis may outperform a non-parametric analysis, by providing less variable results at the expense of a tolerable amount of bias."[1]

Perhaps one of the most common uses for bootstrapping in medical research has been for calculating CIs for derived statistics such as cost-effectiveness ratios, when the theoretical distribution is mathematically difficult although care is needed here since the denominators in some bootstrap samples can get close to 0.

A3.1 Computer analysis

A3.1.1 Two-sample *t*-test with unequal variances

Suppose we wished to compare deadspace in asthmatics and non-asthmatics from the results in Table 2.1. A conventional *t*-test assuming equal variances is given in Table A3.1(i). As described in Chapter 1, this can also be tackled by linear regression as shown in Table A3.1(ii). One can see that the estimated SE of the difference 9.5656 is the same in each case. The difference in means is 30.125 ml and the conventional CI for this difference is 9.46 to 50.79 ml (the estimate is negative for the regression since deadspace is less for asthmatics). Note, however, that the standard deviations are markedly different for the two

Table A3.1 Output illustrating use of the bootstrap to compare two means

(i) Two-sample t-test with equal variances

Group	Obs	Mean	Std. Err.	Std. Dev.	[95% Conf. Interval]	
0	7	83	9.778499	25.87148	59.07287	106.9271
1	8	52.875	2.754461	7.790791	46.36174	59.38826
combined	15	66.93333	6.105787	23.64761	53.83772	80.02894
diff		30.125	9.565644		9.459683	50.79032

Degrees of freedom: 13

Ho: mean(0) - mean(1) = diff = 0

Ha: diff < 0	Ha: diff != 0	Ha: diff > 0
t = 3.1493	t = 3.1493	t = 3.1493
P < t = 0.9962	P > |t| = 0.0077	P > t = 0.0038

(ii) Regression of deadspace against asthma

Deadspce	Coef.	Std. Err.	t	P>|t|	[95% Conf. Interval]	
Asthma	-30.125	9.565644	-3.15	0.008	-50.79032	-9.459683
_cons	83	6.985759	11.88	0.000	67.90819	98.09181

(iii) Bootstrap statistics

Number of obs = 15

Replications = 1000

Variable	Reps	Observed	Bias	Std. Err.	[95% Conf. Interval]	
b_Asthma	1000	-30.125	-572699	9.624754	-49.01205	-11.23795 (N)
					-48	-10.625 (P)
					-46.01786	-7.035714 (BC)
					-44	-3.410714 (BCa)

Note: N = normal
      P = percentile
      BC = bias-corrected
      BCa = bias-corrected and accelerated

groups. One might wish to see how the CI would be changed using a parametric bootstrap. The output from this procedure is given in Table A3.1(iii), which shows four different bootstrap statistics. The BCa bootstrap CI (the recommended one) is 3.4 to 44.0 ml. This is no longer symmetric about the point estimate and the lower end is closer to 0 than the conventional CI estimate.

A3.2 The bootstrap in action

In health economics, Lambert *et al.*[5] calculated the mean resource costs per patient for day patients with active rheumatoid arthritis as £1789 with a bootstrap 95% CI of £1539 to £2027 (1000 replications). They used a bootstrap method because the resource costs have a very skewed distribution. However, the authors did not state which bootstrap method they used.

A3.3 Robust or sandwich estimate SE

The robust or sandwich estimate SE is now a common feature in analyses and is incorporated in many packages. It was first described by Huber[6] and later by White.[7] The terminology is somewhat controversial. It is "robust" in the sense that *if* the model is the one we describe, *except* that the variance is not constant as is normally assumed, *then* the SEs given by the procedure reflect better what we understand by SEs under repeated sampling than those given by the standard model. It is not "robust" in the sense of a non-parametric test, where we can drop a Normality assumption, or if our model for the predictor variable is actually wrong (e.g. if the relationship is not actually linear). It is called the "sandwich" estimator because in matrix notation the estimate brackets either side of a correction factor, thus two pieces of bread with a filling.

Recall that the least squares estimate of β for the model $y_i = \alpha + \beta x_i + \varepsilon_i$ is

$$b = \frac{\sum_{i=1}^{n}(y_i - \bar{y})(x_i - \bar{x})}{\sum_{i=1}^{n}(x_i - \bar{x})^2}.$$

Also recall that for any constants a and b and random variable X, $\mathrm{Var}(aX - b) = a^2\mathrm{Var}(X)$. Thus,

$$\mathrm{Var}(b) = \frac{\sum_{i=1}^{n}\mathrm{Var}(y_i)(x_i - \bar{x})^2}{\left[\sum_{i=1}^{n}(x_i - \bar{x})^2\right]^2}.$$

Conventionally, we assume $\text{Var}(y_i) = \sigma^2$, and so the term $\sum_{i=1}^{n}(x_i - \bar{x})^2$ cancels and we get the usual least squares estimate. However, suppose we were unwilling to assume a constant variance and instead had $\text{Var}(y_i) = \sigma_i^2$. We need an estimate of σ_i^2 and one suggestion is to use the square of the residual e_i. Since σ^2 is usually estimated by $\sum_{i=1}^{n} e_i^2/(n-2)$ we would need to multiply the estimate by $n/(n-2)$ to allow for the fact that a and b are estimates. At first sight one is estimating $n+2$ parameters (the n residuals and the two regression coefficients) with only n data points! However, because the variance is not the main focus of the analysis this procedure turns out to give reasonable estimates. A plot e_i^2 against $(x_i - \bar{x})^2$ will indicate whether a robust estimate will give markedly different results: a positive slope shows that the variance of the residual increases with x, and the robust SE will be bigger than the conventional estimate, a negative slope will indicate the opposite. Robust SEs have also been extended to non-linear models such as logistic regression, but here they are only an approximation and should be used with more caution.

A3.3.1 Example of robust SEs

Consider again the comparison of deadspace in asthmatics and non-asthmatics. As discussed in Swinscow and Campbell[8] (p. 69), if one is in doubt about the equal variance assumption, rather than use a pooled variance estimate, one can combine the variances for each mean to get, $s_1^2/n_1 + s_2^2/n_2$ and adjust the d.f. using either Welch's or Satterthwaite's approximation. This is shown in Table A3.2(i). Note that the P-value of 0.02 is much larger than the 0.0077 obtained assuming equal variances given in Table A3.1. One can obtain the same estimate of the SE using robust regression (Table A3.2(ii), with the HC2 option in STATA to adjust the d.f.). Note, however, the P-value of 0.011 obtained from robust regression assumes a large sample which is not the case here, and so is less than that from the t-test. The main advantage of robust regression is that it fits seamlessly into a regression framework, and so can be used when the number of explanatory variables is more than one. As with the unequal variance t-test, it is less powerful than conventional methods if the assumptions for the model are met, but is better if there is significant heterogeneity of variance. For large samples the loss of efficiency is slight. Note that, in contrast to the bootstrap estimate, the CI is symmetric about the estimate. This is because the robust SE can cope with variance heterogeneity, but not with skewness.

A3.3.2 Uses of robust regression

- In linear regression when there is evidence the variance of the error term is not constant. An alternative here would be to use the bootstrap.

Table A3.2 Computer output using robust regression for unequal variances

(i) Two-sample t-test with unequal variances

Group	Obs	Mean	Std. Err.	Std. Dev.	[95% Conf. Interval]	
0	7	83	9.778499	25.87148	59.07287	106.9271
1	8	52.875	2.754461	7.790791	46.36174	59.38826
combined	15	66.93333	6.105787	23.64761	53.83772	80.02894
diff		30.125	10.15904		6.281123	53.96888

```
Welch's degrees of freedom: 7.26805

                   Ho: mean(0) - mean(1) = diff = 0
Ha: diff < 0              Ha: diff != 0              Ha: diff > 0
   t = 2.9653                 t = 2.9653                 t = 2.9653
P < t = 0.9900        P > |t| = 0.0201           P > t = 0.0100
```

(ii) Regression with robust standard errors

Deadspce	Coef.	Robust HC2 Std. Err.	t	P>|t|	[95% Conf. Interval]	
Asthma	-30.125	10.15904	-2.97	0.011	-52.07227	-8.177728
cons	83	9.778499	8.49	0.000	61.87484	104.1252

- When data are clustered, it is reasonable to assume the variances are the same within clusters, but the data within clusters are correlated (see Chapter 5 for more details).
- To get valid estimates for the SEs of relative risks (see Chapter 6).

A3.4 Reporting the bootstrap and robust SEs in the literature

- State the method of bootstrap used, such as percentile or bias corrected.
- State the number of replications for the bootstrap.
- State what type of robust SE was used.

References

1. Efron B, Tibshirani RJ. *An Introduction to the Bootstrap*. New York: Chapman and Hall, 1993.
2. Davison A, Hinckley D. *Bootstrap Methods and Their Applications*. Cambridge: Cambridge University Press, 1997.

3. Dale G, Fleetwood JA, Weddell A, Elllis RD, Sainsbury JRC. β-endorphin: a factor in "fun-run" collapse. *Br Med J* 1987; **294:** 1004.
4. Altman DG, Machin D, Bryant TN, Gardner MJ, eds. *Statistics with Confidence*, 2nd edn. London: BMJ Books, 2000.
5. Lambert CM, Hurst NP, Forbes JF, Lochhead A, Macleod M, Nuki G. Is day care equivalent to inpatient care for active rheumatoid arthritis? Randomised controlled clinical and economic evaluation. *Br Med J* 1998; **316:** 965–9.
6. Huber PJ. The behaviour of maximum likelihood estimates under non-standard conditions. In: *Proceedings of the Fifth Berkeley Symposium on Mathematical Statistics and Probability*, Vol. 1. Berkeley, CA: University of California Press, 1967: 221–33.
7. White H. A heteroskedasticity-consistent covariance matrix estimator and a direct test for heteroskedasticity. *Econometrika* 1980; **48:** 817–30.
8. Swinscow TDV, Campbell MJ. *Statistics at Square One*, 10th edn. London: BMJ Books, 2002.

Appendix 4 **Bayesian methods**

Consider two clinical trials of equal size for the treatment of headache. One is an analgesic against placebo, and the other is a homoeopathic treatment against placebo. Both give identical P-values (<0.05). Which would you believe? The traditional frequentist approach described in the book does not enable one formally to incorporate beliefs about the efficacy of treatment that one might have held before the experiment, but this can be done using *Bayesian methods*.[1]

Bayes's theorem appeared in a posthumous publication in 1763 by Thomas Bayes, a non-conformist minister from Tunbridge Wells. It gives a simple and uncontroversial result in probability theory, relating probabilities of events before an experiment (*a priori*) to probabilities of events after an experiment (*a posteriori*). The link between the prior and the posterior is the *likelihood*, described in Appendix 2. Specific uses of the theorem have been the subject of considerable controversy for many years and it is only in recent years a more balanced and pragmatic perspective has emerged.[2]

A familiar situation to which Bayes theorem can be applied is diagnostic testing; a doctor's prior belief about whether a patient has a particular disease (based on knowledge of the prevalence of the disease in the community and the patient's symptoms) will be modified by the result of the test.[3] Bayesian methods enable one to make statements such as "the probability that the new treatment is better than the old is 0.95". Under certain circumstances, 95% confidence intervals (CIs) calculated in the conventional (frequentist) manner can be interpreted as "a range of values within which one is 95% certain that the true value of a parameter really lies".[4] Thus it can be argued that a Bayesian approach allows results to be presented in a form that is most suitable for decisions. Bayesian methods interpret data from a study in the light of external evidence and judgement, and the form in which conclusions are drawn contributes naturally to decision-making.[5] Prior plausibility of hypotheses is taken into account, just as when interpreting the results of a diagnostic test. Scepticism about large treatment effects can be formally expressed and used in cautious interpretation of results that cause surprise.

One of the main difficulties with Bayesian methods is the choice of the prior distribution. Different analysts may choose different priors, and so the same data set analysed by different investigators could lead to different conclusions. A commonly chosen prior is an *uninformative prior*, which assigns equal probability to all values over the possible range and leads to analyses that are possibly less subjective than analyses that use priors based on, say, clinical judgement. There are philosophical differences between Bayesians and frequentists, such as the nature of probability, but these should not interfere with a sensible interpretation of data.

A Bayesian perspective leads to an approach to clinical trials that is claimed to be more flexible and ethical than traditional methods.[6]

Bayesian methods do not supplant traditional methods, but complement them. In this book the area of greatest overlap would be in random effects models, described in Chapter 5. Further details are given by Berry and Stangl.[7]

A4.1 Reporting Bayesian methods in the literature[8]

- Report the pre-experiment probabilities and specify how they were determined. In most practical situations, the particular form of the prior information has little influence on the final outcome because it is overwhelmed by the weight of experimental evidence.
- Report the post-trial probabilities and their intervals. Often the mode of the posterior distribution is reported, with the 2.5 and 97.5 centiles (the 95% prediction interval). It can be helpful to plot the posterior distribution.

References

1. Bland JM, Altman DG. Bayesians and frequentists. *Br Med J* 1998; **317:** 1151–2.
2. Spiegelhalter DJ, Myles JP, Jones DR, Abrams KR. Methods in health service research: an introduction to Bayesian methods in health technology assessment. *Br Med J* 1999; **319:** 508–12.
3. Campbell MJ, Machin D. *Medical Statistics: A Commonsense Approach*, 3rd edn. Chichester: John Wiley, 1999.
4. Burton PR, Gurrin LC, Campbell MJ. Clinical significance not statistical significance: a simple Bayesian alternative to *P*-values. *J Epidemiol Commun Health* 1998; **52:** 318–23.
5. Lilford RJ, Braunholtz D. The statistical basis of public policy a paradigm shift is overdue. *Br Med J* 1996; **313:** 603–7.
6. Kadane JB. Prime time for Bayes. *Control Clin Trials* 1995; **16:** 313–18.
7. Berry DA, Stangl DK. *Bayesian Biostatistics*. New York: Marcel Dekker, 1996.
8. Hughes MD. Reporting Bayesian analyses of clinical trials. *Stat Med* 1993; **12:** 1651–63.

Answers to exercises

Chapter 2

1 The assumptions are:
   (i) there is a linear relation between baseline and outcome;
   (ii) acupuncture reduces the number of days of headache irrespective of the baseline value (i.e. treatment effect is the same for all subjects);
   (iii) the residuals from the model are independent and approximately Normally distributed with constant variance.
2 The SD for these data is large relative to the mean, which suggests that in fact the data are likely to be skewed. The data are also restricted to a minimum of 0 and a maximum of 28, which also might lead to skewness. However the mean values are close to centre of the range and sample size is quite large so the P-value is unlikely to be materially changed.
3 The confidence interval for the analysis of covariance is larger than for the t-test. This suggests that there is only a loose association between the baseline and follow-up and so introducing a covariate has actually increased the SE. Note that the numbers of patients at baseline is not the same as that at follow up, so we do not know if those who were followed up were comparable at baseline.
4 One might like to see: a plot of the distribution of the data, a plot of baseline vs follow-up for the two groups as in Figure 2.2 and the baseline values for those actually followed up. One might also like to see if, at baseline, the drop-outs differed from those who were subsequently followed up. A dot plot of the residuals by treatment group would help confirm whether they are plausibly Normally distributed with similar variance in the two groups.

Chapter 3

1 The problems are that the authors have dichotomised a continuous variable and we would like to be reassured that this was done prior to examining

the data. Also dichotomising a continuous variable can result in loss of information. It might lead to a more sensitive analysis if the time to progression was taken into account. Two advantages are: simplicity in summarising the data and that they could combine two outcomes, a continuous one (joint space narrowing) and a discrete one (hip replacement).

2   The increase in the OR for 1 year is 1.06 and so we simply raise this to the power 10 to get the OR as 1.6 in someone 10 years older. It is the same for the 65- vs 75-year-olds – this is a consequence of the model.

3   We have to solve the equation $(\pi/(1 - \pi)/(0.13/0.87)) = 1.8$. This leads to $\pi = 0.21$ or about 21%.

4   The analogous model is Figure 2.3, where the slope with age is linear on the log odds, with different intercepts for males and females.

5   We would expect the model to predict rather fewer than 90%. This is because the parameter were estimated from the same data set as the predictions were made. A better test would be to estimate the model on a subset of the data and make the predictions on the remaining subset.

Chapter 4

Exercise 1
Model 1

1   A = 3 (3 parameters in model); B = 1.10 $(=-2 \times (188.55165 - 188.04719)$); C = -0.487 $(=-0.1512/0.3102)$ Note: It is **not** the ratio of the hazard ratio to its SE. 0.626; D = -0.7592 $(=-0.1512 - 1.96 \times 0.3102)$; E = 0.4568 $(=-0.1512 + 1.96 \times 0.3102)$; F = 0.4580 $(=\exp(-0.7592))$; G = 1.5790 $(=\exp(0.4568))$.

Model 2

1   LR = 10.71, $(=-2 \times (188.0472 - 182.6898))$ d.f. = 4 (4 dummy variables). We find $P = 0.03$, suggesting differences in survival of different histological types.

2   0.763 (95% CI 0.272 to 0.214).

3   $(0.9978)^{10} = 0.9782$.

Exercise 2

1   A stratified analysis was used because the authors wished to allow for possible differences in the ages of the exposed and non-exposed groups, but did not wish to assume a particular model for age. A stratified analysis assumes the risk is the same for each person within a 10-year age cohort, and that this risk may vary as the cohort ages. However, a person within a different 10-year cohort may have a different risk profile as they age. The

fact that the hazard ratio changes little when smoking is included in the model suggests that the groups are well matched for smoking habit. The fact that the hazard is reduced when FEV1 is included suggests that perhaps the slate workers were already suffering with a low FEV1 at baseline, and so FEV1 and slate exposure are not independent covariates. Two major assumptions in model 2 are the proportional hazards assumption, which means that the risk of slate exposure remains constant over the 24 years, and a lack of interaction assumption, which means the effect of slate is the same whether of not the man is a smoker. The former could be examined by the log–log survival plot as described in Chapter 4 and the latter by fitting interaction terms in the model. The interpretation of the coefficient associated with FEV1, is that for two people who are in the same 10-year age group, exposure category and smoking category, one with an FEV1 l greater than the other has a risk of death of 74% compared to the other.

Chapter 5

1 Difference in means is 0.42.
2 Weights are: Treatment 1: 0.22, 0.22, 0.19, 0.24, 0.22; Treatment 2: 0.22, 0.22, 0.22, 0.22, 0.22. Difference in means is 0.39.
3 Difference in means is 0.41.
4 Note that (1) is given by the robust SE method, (2) is given approximately by the maximum likelihood and gee method, and (3) is given by the summary measures method.
There seems to some evidence that treatment 2 has more variability between practices and practice 6 appears to be an outlier which might be investigated.

Chapter 6

1 (i) The potential confounders were categorised so that the investigators could count the number of events and the exposure time in each category. If any of the confounders were continuous, then the number of events would be 0 or 1. (ii) In fact the model is a *log-linear* one so one would expect a plot of the *log* of the incidence rates to be linearly related to the birth weight. In practice it might be difficult to distinguish between a linear and a log plot. (iii) One could examine whether the data were overdispersed and if so, the SEs would need adjustment. (iv) Since time from birth to a diagnosis of diabetes is like a survival time one could employ Cox regression as described in Chapter 4.
2 The main outcome is an ordinal variable since we can assume that "too early" is a response between "at the right age" and "should not have happened"

but we cannot assign ranks to these categories. Thus we could use ordinal regression. It would be better than logistic regression because it does not require a dichotomy in the outcome, and if the assumptions are met, will prove to be more powerful. A multivariate model is necessary to see if the outcome is affected by confounders such as social class and parenting style. The main assumption is one of proportional odds between the categories and the authors state they checked this. Without allowing for covariates this could be checked informally as follows. For girls the percentages in the 3 groups are 55;32;13 and for boys they are 68;25;5. Pooling the second and third categories the percentages are 55;45 for girls and 68;30, and pooling the first and second they are 87;13 and 95;5. The odds for girls compared to boys of being "at right age" vs the other categories is (0.55/0.45)/(0.68/0.32) = 0.58. The odds for "at right age" or "too early" vs "should not have happened" is (0.87/0.13)/(0.95/0.05) = 0.35. These are both in the same direction but not particularly close and based on the discussion in Chapter 6 and the reassurances from the authors of the papers one might be happy that the assumption is met.

Glossary

Analysis of variance (ANOVA)   A form of linear model with a continuous outcome variable and categorical input variables.

Analysis of covariance (ANCOVA)   A form of linear model with a continuous outcome variable, some categorical input variables and usually just one continuous input variable.

Autoregressive model   A model for a time dependent outcome variable which in which the error term includes past values of itself.

Bayesian methods   Methods which allow parameters to have distributions. Initially the parameter θ is assigned a prior distribution $P(\theta)$, and after data, X, have been collected a posterior distribution $P(\theta|X)$ is obtained using *Bayes' Theorem*, which links the two via the **likelihood** $P(X|\theta)$.

Binary variable   A variable which can take only two values, say "success" and "failure".

Binomial distribution   The distribution of a **binary variable** when the probability of a "success" is constant.

Bootstrap   A computer intensive resampling method to calculate standard errors without relying on model assumptions.

Censored data   An observation is censored at X if all we know is that the observation is $\geq X$. Often used with survival data, where all we know is that a subject has survived X amount of time.

Cluster randomised trial   A trial in which the subjects are randomised in clusters.

Cochrane–Orcutt method   A method of removing **serial correlation** in regression models.

Complementary log–log transform   If $0 < P < 1$ then the transform is $\log_e[-\log(1 - P)]$. Used as an alternative to the **logit transform** in **logistic regression**.

Conditional logistic regression   Used to analyse binary data from matched case–control studies, or from cross-over trials.

Continuation ratio model   A form of **ordinal regression model**. Suppose we have a 3 level ordinal outcome and a binary explanatory variable. If p_1,

p_2 and $p_3 = 1 - p_1 - p_2$ are the probabilities of a subject being in levels 1, 2 or 3 when the explanatory variable is at one value and q_1, q_2 and $q_3 = 1 - q_1 - q_2$ are the probabilities of a subject being in levels 1, 2 or 3 when the explanatory variable is the other value. Then the model assumes $[p_2/(p_1 + p_2)]/[q_1/(q_1 + q_2)] = p_3/q_3$.

Design effect (**DE**)   The amount that a variance of an estimator has to be inflated to allow for clustering, or other aspects of the sampling scheme.

Dummy variables   Binary variables used for fitting categorical terms, in which each dummy takes the value 0 or 1, and if there are n categories, there are $n - 1$ independent dummy variables.

Durbin–Watson test   A test for **serial correlation** in a time series.

Deviance   A measure of how far a set of data varies from a perfect fit to a model. For Normally distributed residuals it is equal to the residual sum of squares.

Effect modification   Given a model with an input variable and an outcome, effect modification occurs if the observed relationship is changed markedly when a third variable is included in the model. An extreme example of this is **Simpson's paradox.**

Extra-Binomial or extra-Poisson variation   This occurs when the variation in the data, allowing for the covariates, is greater than would be predicted by the Binomial (or Poisson) distribution.

Fixed effect   A term in a model that can be fitted using **dummy variables.** The assumption is that if a new set of data were to be collected, the population parameter would be the same (fixed). Thus the effect of an intervention in a trial is assumed fixed.

Forest plot   A plot used in **meta-analysis**. Usually it comprises a series of estimates and confidence intervals from the component studies, and a summary estimate and confidence interval. Supposedly named because it appears like a set of trees.

Funnel plot   A plot used in **meta-analysis** to try and detect **publication bias.** It comprises a plot of the precision of estimates of treatment effects from component studies vs the estimate itself.

Generalised estimating equations (**gee**)   A set of equations for estimating parameters in a model, essentially equal to iteratively re-weighted **least squares**. They are commonly used with a **sandwich estimator** to obtain the standard error. There is also **GEE2** includes the variance estimators in the set of equations.

Hazard rate   The probability per time unit that a case that has survived to the beginning of the respective interval will fail in that interval. Specifically, it is computed as the number of failures per time units in the respective interval, divided by the average number of surviving cases at the mid-point of the interval.

Hazard ratio (**Relative hazard**)   Hazard ratio compares two groups differing in treatments or prognostic variables, etc. If the hazard ratio is 2.0, then the rate of failure in one group is twice the rate in the other group. Can be interpreted as a **relative risk.**

Hosmer–Lemeshow statistic   A measure of the goodness-of-fit of a **logistic regression** when at least one of the explanatory variables is continuous.

Influential points   In regression analysis, points which, if deleted and the model refitted, would have a big effect on at least one of the model parameters.

Kaplan–Meier plot   An empirical plot of the probability of survival on the y-axis by survival time on the x-axis. Censored observations can be incorporated in the plot.

Least-squares   A method of estimating parameters in a model when the outcome is continuous. It fits a linear model by minimising the residual sum of squares. *Weighted least squares* applies weights to the residuals, usually the inverse of a variance estimate. *Iteratively reweighted least squares* allows the weights to vary depending on the current fitted values and so requires iteration to be solved.

Leverage points   In regression analysis, observations that have an extreme value on one or more explanatory variable. The leverage values indicate whether or not X values for a given observation are outlying (far from the main body of the data). They may be **influential points.**

Likelihood   The probability of a set of observations given a model. If the model has a single parameter θ, it is denoted $P(X|\theta)$, where X denotes the data.

Likelihood ratio test   A general purpose test of model M_0 against an alternative M_1 where M_0 is contained within M_1. It is based on the ratio of two likelihood functions one derived from each of H_0 and H_1. The statistics $-2\,ln$ (L_{M_0}/L_{M_1}) has approximately a Chi-square distribution with d.f. equal to the difference in the number of parameters in the two models.

Linear model   A model which is linear in the parameters, but not necessarily in the variables. Thus $y = \beta_0 + \beta_1 X + \beta_2 X^2$ is a linear model but $y = \exp(\beta_0 + \beta_1 X)$ is not.

Logit transform   If $0 < P < 1$ then $logit(P) = \log_e[P/(1 - P)]$. When the outcome is binary, often also called the **logistic** transform.

Logistic regression   Used to analyse data where the outcome variable is **binary**. It uses the **logistic** transform of the expected probability of "success".

Maximum likelihood   A method of fitting a model by choosing parameters that maximises the **likelihood** of the data.

Meta-analysis   A method of combining results from different studies to produce a overall summary statistic, usually in clinical trials.

Mixed model   A model that mixes **random** and **fixed effect** terms.

Multiple linear regression   Often just known as **multiple regression**. Used to analyse data when the outcome is continuous and the model is **linear.**

Odds   If p_1 is the probability of a success, the odds is the ratio of the probability of a success to a failure $p_1/(1 - p_1)$.

Odds ratio   Used as a summary measure for binary outcomes. If p_1 is the probability of a success in one group and p_2 the probability of success in another, then the odds ratio is $[p_1/(1 - p_1)]/[p_2/(1 - p_2)]$.

Ordinal variable   A categorical variable, where the categories can be ordered, such as pain scores of "mild", "moderate" and "severe".

Ordinal regression   Used to analyse data when the outcome variable is ordinal. Usually uses the **proportional odds** model or the **continuation ratio** model.

Over-dispersion   In a Poisson and Binomial model, the variance of the outcome is determined by the mean value. When the observed value exceeds this predicted value, the data are said to be overdispersed. This can happen when the counts are correlated.

Poisson distribution   The distribution of a count variable when the probability of an event is constant.

Poisson regression   Used to analyse data when the outcome variable is a count.

Proportional hazards model (*also* the **Cox** model)   Used to analyse survival data. The main assumption is if an explanatory variable is binary, then the **hazard ratio** for this variable is constant over time.

Proportional odds model   Used when outcome is ordinal. Suppose we have an ordinal outcome with 3 categories and a binary explanatory variable. A proportional odds model assumes that the odds ratio for the outcome variable comparing levels 1 and 2 of the outcome is the same as the odds ratio for the outcome variable comparing levels 2 and 3.

Publication bias   A phenomenon when some studies which have been conducted fail to be published. It usually occurs because studies that have positive findings are more likely to be written up and submitted for publication, and editors are more likely to accept them.

Random effects model   A model with more than one random (or error) term. The assumption is that if the study was done again, the terms would estimate different population parameters, in contrast to a **fixed effects** model. Thus in a longitudinal study, the effect of a patient on the intervention effect is assumed random.

Relative risk   Used as a summary measure for binary outcomes for prospective studies. If p_1 is the probability of success in one group and p_2 the probability of success in another, the relative risk is p_1/p_2. If p_1 and p_2 are the incidences of an event, then the relative risk is also the **incidence rate ratio**.

Robust standard error (*also* **sandwich estimator**)   A method of estimating standard errors of parameters without assuming the error variances are homogenous.

Sandwich estimator   A robust standard error, so-called because the matrix formulation is like a "sandwich" ABA, where A is the "bread" and B the "filling".

Score test   A measure of the fit of a set of parameters to a model, based of the slope of the likelihood of the data of model at the null point.

Serial correlation (*also* **autocorrelation**)   In time series when values of a variable are correlated in time.

Simpson's paradox   This occurs when one has binary input and output variables and a third variable which is related to both. When a model is fitted that does not include the third variable the observed relationship between the input and output variables is in one direction, and when the third variable is included in the model the direction of the relationship is reversed.

Stepwise regression   Used to decide which of a set of explanatory variables best describes the outcome. Also includes step-up and step-down regression where variables are progressively added or subtracted from the model.

Time series regression   Regression in which the outcome variable is time dependent.

Wald test   A measure of the fit of a parameter of a model based on the estimate of the parameter divided by its estimated standard error.

Weibull distribution   A parametric distribution for survival data.

Index